A PELVIC FLOOR DIALOGUE

A PELVIC FLOOR DIALOGUE

ILLNESS, METAPHOR AND HEALING

Lorraine Liebowitz-Mann

Quickfox

Published by Quickfox Publishing
PO Box 494 Howard Place 7450
Cape Town, South Africa
www.quickfox.co.za | info@quickfox.co.za

A Pelvic Floor Dialogue: Illness, Metaphor and Healing
ISBN 978-0-620-76646-3

First edition 2017

www.pelvicfloordialogue.co.za

Edited by Rachel Bey-Miller
Proofread by Nadine Dove
Book and cover design by Vanessa Wilson
Typesetting and production by Quickfox Publishing
Printing by Digital Action SA, Cape Town

To my granddaughter,
Adi

ACKNOWLEDGEMENTS

To my elder daughter, Yael, for her steadfastness throughout the journey and for providing me with a safe place to land. Your strength and support meant the world to me. You walked those corridors of hope and despair with me. Remain the matriarch and healer that you are.

To my younger daughter Elisheva, for being there in caring ways that made the journey that much easier. You took over the immediate realms of care and remained steadfast. Never lose sight of who you were meant to be.

To my granddaughter, Adi, for all the many discourses around life, death, hopes, dreams and fears that we shared. No topic was too painful, no corner left unexplored. Thank you for your companionship, deep wisdom and love. I'll remember to send you a sign.

To Gwen, for saving a soul. Everyone should have one such friend in this world.

To Nanette, my compass, my comfort, for providing me with a sacred healing space in which to share the unspoken grief and truths of the cost of the journey, sans judgement.

To Rachel, my Hindu Other, for her unwavering friendship and potent dialogues concerning purpose, suffering and meaning. You never gave up on me or stopped believing in my potential. The catalyst for my extraordinary journey into the realm of the Spirit and true healing.

To all of you who made the difference,
I thank you

A special thank you to my publishing dream team:
Vanessa Wilson of Quickfox Publishing for layout, typesetting, design and advice
Rachel Bey-Miller for writing advice and editing
Nadine Dove for content reviewing and proofreading

CONTENTS

PART 2 | PATIENT GUIDE

MOTIVATION FOR WRITING THIS BOOK

This book serves as a resource for patients undergoing and recovering from pelvic floor[1] surgery. It addresses the numerous quality-of-life shifts associated with pelvic floor surgery, exploring its inherent challenges and losses. It opens a discourse on a hitherto taboo subject for the many women who have suffered in silence over the years. It affords a glimpse into one woman's life, who upon exiting from the confines of the medical structures of care, undertakes to explore the human cost of illness on many levels (spiritual, physical, emotional, and social), and the courage and resilience required along the way. It provides a glimpse into her personal story from health to shades of physical, emotional and spiritual healing. It explores the notion that illness can be viewed as a gift, an invitation to transform, to choose another life. It speaks of healing on many levels, and the role forgiveness plays in the journey to health.

1 The network of tissues, ligaments and muscles that support the organs in the pelvis, including the uterus, vagina, bladder and rectum

This is an informative read for multi-disciplinary personnel in the field of pelvic floor syndrome. It is a must-read for those who are ill, yet are willing to entertain the possibility that illness is a gift, a catalyst for a life not yet born; an invitation to recommit to life, albeit in a different way. It is a story of inner transformation, the soul's work, which needs urgent attention during the onslaught of illness.

Notes

See *Part 2, Chapter 1: Signs and symptoms of pelvic floor dysfunction* for illustrated descriptions of the various types of prolapse and incontinence experienced by women with this condition.

As a patient or someone suspecting that you have pelvic floor dysfunction of some kind, please refer to:

http://www.uchospitals.edu/specialties/pelvic/faq/index.html

http://www.mayoclinic.org/diseases-conditions/pelvic-organ-prolapse/in-depth/transvaginal-mesh-complications/art-20110300

PRELUDE

Meeting Lorraine over twenty years ago was like meeting someone deeply known, cut from the same soul cloth. That instantaneous recognition of an ancient bond has been active and nurtured ever since. Our lives and experiences are very different, but the difference has never become a barrier because the bond has always remained a bridge.

We have witnessed one another's struggles and successes; we have shared books and laughter; we have been the best of loyal friends. And in more recent years I have been her witness in a caring warzone, where surgeons and others did and still do what they can with what they have. But what if there is massive scarring from previous battles? How do you stitch a scar to a scar? You do, in the vain hope that it will hold.

This is not an easy read. There is not much obvious beauty here. A beautiful soul, yes, but not a beautiful story. Neither is it a fairy tale. There can't be fairy tales about women over 50 whose only sin was to bear children the old-fashioned way.

Childbirth is a sanctified subject in our society. The damage it wreaks is never discussed. Hysterectomies are a dime a dozen. What happens in the hollow they leave behind? Never discussed.

To pillage Yeats[2], things fall apart, the centre cannot hold. He certainly didn't intend to describe prolapse, fissures, tears and other unspeakable female problems, but this is how these women feel – that things are falling apart and the centre cannot hold. And no one speaks about it. There is no patient narrative out there, and certainly no patient guide to explain how things fall apart and what to expect next.

In this book, Lorraine breaks the silence – the silence of our mothers – and brings us strange beauty and hidden transformations. She brings hope to those whose deepest wounding speaks to their highest good...their ability to nurture even as they struggle.

May this book be a blessing for them.

Rachel Bey-Miller
April 2017 | Cape Town

---

2 Torn from *The Second Coming* by William Butler Yeats

Journal entry 25.12.2016

My first visit to Jerusalem was in 1968, aged 16. I returned in 1974, aged 22, as a married woman and spent a year studying in a Yeshiva[3], an experience I found profoundly enriching and stimulating. In 1983, I returned with my two daughters and their father, departing again in 1986. We resided in Gilo, a small suburb on the outskirts of Jerusalem, once part of the occupied territory taken during the Six Day War.

Being a relatively new suburb, it boasted a vibrant young population and numerous kindergartens, reflective of a flourishing new generation. Down the road from Gilo, if you turned to the right at the T-junction, you would make your way to Bethlehem. If you turned left, you would find yourself driving past olive tree orchards as you wound your way towards the Old City of Jerusalem. Near our apartment was an Absorption Centre for Olim Chadashim[4], and this is where I spent the first six months in Israel learning to speak Hebrew.

Today, three decades later, on this cold, overcast winter day, I find myself once again in Jerusalem, with my elder daughter, her husband and their children, Tal and Adi. We drive slowly towards the Old City. We park and then carefully wind our way down the ancient, cobble-stone streets, flanked by street vendors and snuggled quaint shops, heading towards the Kottel, known to many as the Wailing Wall. The smells of familiar foods permeate the air, the spices of old, lingering as you pass; colourful wares catching my eye along the way. Soon we arrive at a military checkpoint, and once through, my eyes fall upon the Kottel. I stand quietly to the

3 Theological seminary

4 Newly arrived immigrants

side for a long time, just taking it all in, then slowly descend the steps and hesitantly make my way towards the women's section.

Women are huddled together praying, some with an intensity that shakes their small frames. Others are seated. Several women and young girls are leaving, and many of them are walking backwards, as is the custom when one leaves this holy site. I find a seat close to the Mechitzah[5] and sit down. The ambience is electric and I sit riveted, taking in the beauty of the Jerusalem stone, the doves perched in crannies and the odd branch growing from the crevices, reminding us that even as nature abhors a vacuum, it defaults to health and growth.

This is no ordinary visit. I had been in bed for three days prior, exhausted from the endless walking around Tel Aviv and Jaffa in my seventh year of living with pelvic floor complications, having had five surgeries in the last six years. The journey has taken its toll, leaving me quite depleted. I ponder upon the fact that this is my last trip to the Kottel.

Suddenly tears surface, and roll down my cheeks as my lips start to utter a prayer. It is significant from my perspective, being at this sacred site in the autumn years of my life. For this I am very grateful. I begin to thank Hashem[6] for the journey He has sent my soul on during this lifetime; for the opportunities and challenges that have been sent my way, small or big, manageable or difficult. I thank for the illness that has accompanied me over the years, that has brought me to a place where I can offer this prayer with humility.

For myself, there is little to ask for. It is time to realise that I have walked the journey with Him at my side, and the knowing

5 A divider separating men and women in prayer

6 The Name/G-d

that He will be there when I take my last breath. I ask for insight to make the right decisions going forward and for an easy passing when the time is right. I acknowledge that I will not return to this place again in this form, and that He is the only constant in my life. I appeal to Him to guard over my loved ones on the road ahead.

And then I sit for a while before raising my weary body, slowly shuffling backward, to re-enter the three-dimensional reality of modern Jerusalem. But I leave shalem – at peace and with a feeling of completion.

PART 1

My Story

CHAPTER ONE

THE FIRE IN THE BELLY

> *Illness is the night side of life, a more onerous citizenship. Everyone who is born holds dual citizenship, in the kingdom of the well and in the kingdom of the sick. Although we all prefer to use the good passport, sooner or later each of us is obliged, at least for a spell, to identify ourselves as citizens of that other place.*
>
> SUSAN SONTAG

Q You have taken it upon yourself to share your narrative in book form. Are there any thoughts that come to mind concerning your personal narrative?

It is through the retelling of narratives that patients establish a new normality. My story is an intimate one, reflecting on that private place inhabited by women and partnered by surgeons. The narrative explores the complex journey of a life lived in health, then nibbled away by dis-ease and finally ravaged by pelvic floor dysfunction over a period of six years.

Illness forced me to find a way to reintegrate the fragments of a life once known. For me, it symbolises a place where every facet of my life came under scrutiny and stringent review.

Carolyn Myss's words resonated for me. She talks of illness being the catalyst for transformation, an invitation to take on a different citizenship with a different worldview born of struggle. She acknowledges that no matter how healthy we may feel at any given moment, there will inevitably come a time in each of our lives when we are called to be healed. She describes the vulnerability that arises at these times as "that feeling of waiting on the edge of hope or hopelessness that few other conditions in life can activate within us. The vulnerability comes from the disruption of the life force itself." It is associated with a feeling of energy leakage, often experienced by the patient as a dance with health and illness, life and death.

On a deeper psychological level, I have come to view illness as a metaphor for unexpressed suffering. This allows for a more compassionate version of my story, reflecting the relationship between early wounding and the body's reflection of it. Jonathan Kabbat Zinn speaks of the need to respond to the metaphor of our symptoms in such a way as to decipher the unconscious messages our body, psyche and mind wish to impart to us. It serves as a signpost pointing us toward the unexamined, unexplored parts of ourselves; those very parts in need of acknowledgement, rectification and healing. It begs an end to the punishing self-talk and destructive narratives that robbed us of becoming who we were rightfully meant to be and were becoming.

Life and the journey are processes and only when identified, lived to the full and explored without boundaries, will they ensure me the privilege to peek in on the slivers of jewels waiting to be identified, acknowledged and revealed, in the hope that they will be used to reach my ultimate destination.

Q What did you hope to highlight in the narrative of the book?

Research in the area of pelvic floor syndrome has failed to provide rich, soulful narratives into the quality-of-life shifts for women undergoing pelvic floor surgery and recovery. Confronted with repeated pelvic floor surgeries over a six-year period, it was disconcerting to me that there was no narrative to turn to as a reference; no guidelines, no markers along the way. There is a need for a commitment to break the silence around this unspoken pandemic in women's health.

While I am acutely aware that each journey into illness and reclaimed health is unique to the person undertaking it, common themes will and do occur. Failing to highlight the impact of illness on the lived experiences of patients and their families marginalises patients' illness narration.

This book provides an opportunity to explore the purpose, meaning and experience of illness over time. That illness serves as a disruption of the life force goes without saying. It is relentless in its onslaught and can be ruthless in its impact. And it takes great courage and wisdom to accept the condition, the changes it brings, and the many compromises and adaptations it demands along the way. This is not a journey for the faint of heart. In this challenge, the patient is invited to explore the meaning of their life, the purpose of their illness and the many unanswered questions that may surface.

For me, the journey was one of review, rectification, acceptance and redirection. Most of the work remained invisible to the naked eye. To all intents and purposes, this may appear fragmented on the outside, but the inner work becomes a tapestry far more beautiful and complex than it was before the onset of the illness. It exposes unanswered questions never explored with the same intensity, precisely because chronic illness forces you to confront your own mortality. And this is a very humbling and sobering challenge to undertake. It begs for a life review before and after the onset of illness, and may be the trigger for confronting compromised quality of life going forward, if not mortality.

I realised in hindsight that there is much that can be achieved despite the onslaught of illness and during the time of adversity. In its own unique way the experience of illness over a six-year period was a gift that taught me the value of review and reintegration of one's lived experiences. Through the synthesis, there was value in the journey, far more profound than I would ever have anticipated. Narration of my personal journey will hopefully provide the reader with more clarity on why I regard illness as a gift, an opportunity for transformation.

And so, my story begins…

The issues of incomplete bladder excretion and associated bladder infections date back to early childhood. In 1963, aged 11, I underwent a bladder stretch owing to a congenital narrowing of the urethra.

In 1983, while living in Israel, I presented with severe rectal bleeding. I was referred to a surgeon who upon examination reported a large fissure and suggested that this be attended to under a local anaesthetic. On the day of the procedure, I was asked to kneel in a foetal position while the surgeon anaesthetised the area and proceeded to attend to the stretching of the anal passage. Upon completion of the procedure, my body went into shock. I began to shake so uncontrollably that I had to be assisted in dressing. I returned home to recuperate.

In 1990, at the age of 38, I underwent a hysterectomy for uterine prolapse in conjunction with a bladder lift for bladder stress incontinence.

In 1996, I was referred to a surgeon whose findings showed an anterior mucosal prolapse and an irritable bowel. I was referred to Groote Schuur Hospital for a flexible sigmoidoscopy.

In 2002, I was once again referred to a surgeon who reported changed bowel movements, a right iliac mass and haemorrhoids. The colonoscopy was incomplete due to the inability to get past the hepatic flexure. Removal of the haemorrhoids causing the bleeding proved to be successful.

In 2006, aged 54, I collapsed in my apartment one evening and was rushed off to hospital by ambulance. I was diagnosed with hypertension and put on medication. I developed a persistent cough in the weeks that followed. I was diagnosed with asthma and was twice admitted to Emergency Room outpatients for difficulty in breathing.

This carried on for a year, and with it surfaced pelvic pain. I returned to the pulmonologist for a check-up, only to be reassured that my diagnosis of asthma was in fact incorrect and that the year-long struggle with coughing was a side-effect of the hypertension medication. Withdrawal of the medication addressed the constriction in my chest, only to be replaced by discomfort and pain in the pelvic area coupled with a feeling of something stuck or protruding out of my vagina.

If it was not happening at one end, it was beginning to happen at another, I thought. The damage had been done.

Q What is your understanding of why you were so confused about the symptoms you were experiencing at the time?

All my life, I had diligently attended to my physical health and birthed two children with relative ease. I was prepared for the hormonal changes that surface in midlife. But I had no reference point for the feeling of pressure and bloating in my abdomen.

The first realisation I came to was that there were certain areas in women's health that were taboo, even amongst women. This was a profound realisation.

I understood that women did not discuss their bowel and voiding concerns at tea parties. If their discussions were ever reflective of pelvic floor as a women's issue, then clearly it was a rare occurrence. But statistics did not support this. It is estimated that pelvic floor disorders affect roughly 25% of women in the age group 30–70 worldwide, and that by 2030, more than one fifth of women will present with prolapse after the age of 50. Eleven percent of these patients will require surgery, with a 30–50% failure rate, compromising their quality of life.

Once again, it begs the question, "Why the silence?"

» What on earth was the conspiracy of silence all about?
» Why were we isolated in our sisterhood?

- » Why had I never been educated about pelvic floor at my yearly gynaecological visits?
- » Why all the secrecy about this aspect of women's health?

According to Brené Brown, a well-known shame researcher, shame needs three things to grow exponentially in our lives: secrecy, silence and judgement. For the most part and for too long, women have remained largely uneducated concerning the prevalence and symptoms associated with pelvic organ prolapse (POP). I realised that these concerns and the silence surrounding them would not be easily broken for a multitude of reasons, among them culture, gender, patriarchy, discrimination and shame. It is a systemic conspiracy in its complexity, and the very nature of the conspiracy does not serve the health of women suffering in silence, nor their health-seeking behaviour and required early intervention.

The conspiracy of silence has systemic knock-on effects. There is a distinct lack of population-based epidemiological studies on pelvic floor syndrome, a lack of national statistics on its prevalence combined with a lack of funding for research in this field of women's health. The lack of research in the field is matched only by the dearth of specialists who are trained in this complex field of surgery.

Lack of qualitative research studies precludes women from having an opportunity to narrate the biopsychosocial impact of pelvic floor syndrome on their lives. The stark absence of advocacy work in this field is of concern, as is the lack of public education, for women in particular, on the inherent risks of being a future statistic requiring an intervention. The lack of patient narrative failed to highlight the needs of these patients and the support they required. The net result is that patients remain voiceless.

Q Would you mind sharing your journey towards your diagnosis?

I came across a quote by Dr Seuss that made me smile because it reminded me of the lengths I had to go to be diagnosed correctly.

> *You'll get mixed up, of course, as you already know.*
> *You'll get mixed up with many strange birds as you go.*
> *So be sure when you step. Step with care and great tact*
> *and remember that Life's a Great Balancing Act.*
> *Just never forget to be dexterous and deft.*
> *And never mix up your right foot with your left.*

It is amazing the lengths people go to when they feel desperate. You feel like the life force is leaving you and you don't have a diagnosis to explain it. Unashamedly, I consulted a medium who came highly recommended. Clearly there were some things that women did talk about! Being a novel experience for me, I listened with curiosity as she rambled on while I diligently took notes. Then the following words came out of her mouth:

"Your father says that you are about to undergo major surgery and your parents are worried about this. They say that it must be done, but caution you not to rush into it. If you are not comfortable with the first person, then find another. The sooner you do it the better because it will be less traumatic. You are cautioned to use your intuition and to be comfortable with the surgeon undertaking the procedure. Your father says that the man who will do the surgery is the best at what he does. Your mother warns you that the surgery has to be done."

The news left me feeling overwhelmed and with difficulty I concentrated on the remainder of the session. To be truthful, I was in utter shock.

In search of a diagnosis

I went home and immediately made an appointment to see a urologist. A few days later, I sat opposite him, desperate to find an answer to my recurrent bladder infections and pelvic pain. I shared that at the age of eleven, I had undergone a bladder stretch owing to a congenital narrowing of the urethra. After taking a brief history and clarifying the presenting symptoms, the urologist continued to administer several tests.

"Please bear down," he requested. As I did so, he suggested that there might be something I was not telling him. I did not know what he was referring to.

"Do you have trouble related to bowel functioning?" he asked. And slowly the puzzle was beginning to make sense.

So the pelvic floor pressure was related to an actual condition. I nodded in the affirmative. The examination revealed that the central perineal[7] tendon was not intact, and that a Grade I cystocele[8] and the beginning stages of a rectocele[9] were present. It was noted that I suffered from combined stress and urinary incontinence.

He assured me that both prolapses could be rectified surgically when the condition became more marked. He prescribed a three-month course of antibiotics and probiotics, and requested that I return for a check-up at the end of this period.

I was gobsmacked. Clearly, I had not sufficiently relayed the anguish I had been experiencing every day for some years now. I

---

7 The perineum is generally defined as the surface region between the pubic bone at the front and the coccyx at the base of the spine.

8 A condition in which the wall between the bladder and the vagina weakens to the point that the bladder bulges (prolapses) into the vagina

9 A condition in which the wall between the rectum and the vagina weakens to the point that the rectum bulges (prolapses) into the vagina

felt like I was a malingerer and this small problem-and-treatment option confirmed that. I drove to the pharmacy and picked up the script, my father's words still ringing in my ears. I began to experience a deep sense of foreboding. I feared that no one would be able to diagnose with accuracy the daily onslaught of pain and suffering I was experiencing.

In search of a second opinion

Not satisfied with the first diagnosis, I opted for a second opinion. I booked a flight to Cape Town to see my gynaecologist, who noted a bulge in my abdominal area and the early stages of a rectocele.

Surgical intervention was not indicated at this early stage. He suggested manual manipulation. I remained silent, but secretly thought to myself, as I listened in total disbelief, "Not in your lifetime or mine."

In my humble opinion, these doctors had simply followed the path of least resistance as reflected in the saying, "When you hear hoof beats, think horses not zebras." But this was my life and this was their diagnosis, and thankfully I had the sense to continue the search for an accurate diagnosis.

I had heard of a medical practitioner who specialised in dietetics and made an appointment to see her. It was an unusual experience in that she seemed more interested in me as a human being than the few kilos that needed to be shed. Some may have referred to her as old school, but old school certainly worked for me. It brought back memories of my childhood, when doctors did home visits and mothers kept one in bed for a cold.

When I shared my concerns with her, she suggested that I see her brother, a professor of gynaecology in Johannesburg. She was convinced that I required a surgical intervention, and assured me the he could do the operation with his eyes closed – such was her confidence in him. Thanks to her intervention, I could see him within a week.

Symptoms have a narrative of their own, and had any of them been curious or thorough enough, I would not be seeing a fourth specialist in the space of six weeks, still not accurately diagnosed.

Most patients may have accepted the first diagnosis, and continued to live their lives in quiet desperation, ceding their right to treatment to a higher authority. I found this alarming.

Meeting the truthteller

I waited for two hours to see the professor of gynaecology. He was known to spend quality time with his patients, so no one seemed to mind the wait. As I entered the room, I felt a strange sense of ease and knew that this appointment would be a turning point of sorts. I explained why I had made the appointment, and provided relevant background information related to previous surgeries. Following a vaginal and rectal examination – that was a first! – he sat down on a stool beside the examination table.

I watched his pursed lips and concerned expression, and realised that something serious was wrong. He proceeded to tell me that I had a "gaping wound" inside me, and that I required a major surgical intervention. He felt ill-equipped to undertake the surgery, and referred me to a highly respected colleague at the colorectal unit. He added, in passing, that sexual expression would not be possible following surgery of this magnitude.

Validation at last – the symptoms were not all in my head. It reminded me of the hypochondriac's tombstone: I told you I was sick!

I met with the colorectal surgeon to discuss my diagnosis and consider available options. Initially, he opted for the conservative route, which involved referral to a physiotherapist for pressure point release and Biofeedback.

But once the MRI and defaecogram results were out, it was clear that surgery was the best way forward. I felt relieved that a decision had finally been reached and that health was on its way. I also felt that surgery would be the catalyst for a new life. And it was, but it had little to do with the life I had envisaged post-surgery, and would take years of ongoing adaptation. The surgeon's words still lingered in my ears: "I can heal you structurally, but I cannot take the pain away."

What a strange comment, I thought when I left. But it was to prove to be profound. What I did not realise at the time was that this surgery would invite healing into my life on a multitude of levels. Yes, he could heal me structurally through surgery. He knew that structural repair would not heal my physical pain. But what he did not know was that structural healing would be the catalyst for me to undertake a journey to explore a pain far more riveting that physical pain. I was ill and I needed to heal, but what this would entail only became clear to me in hindsight.

Connecting the dots: end of the road – beginning of the journey

From the outset, the narrative of illness brought with it disruption of my daily life. The sick role accompanied by the blue examination gowns, seemed to draw up new boundaries on all fronts. Predictable work schedules now had to accommodate the pre-operative workup. The tests were many and varied. Some dignified, others less so. Time had to be scheduled for various tests, doctors' visits and physiotherapy. The simple ones involved no more intrusiveness than the filling out of a medical questionnaire related to urinary and faecal incontinence.

The defaecogram shuffle

Dynamic defaecography is a procedure used to evaluate the pelvic floor and rectum while the patient is having a bowel movement. It is commonly referred to as a defaecogram and was by far the most invasive procedure I had to endure. In case you think I am exaggerating, bear with me (excuse the pun) while I entertain you with this unusual test, which was to be repeated several times in the years ahead.

Patiently I type "defaecogram" into Google, but even the Internet has gone silent, such is the shame associated with the arse-end of the world. So let me try the layman's test and describe it in words only you would understand.

A day before the procedure, you are requested to take Precoprep[10] to empty your bowels. This cocktail is an acquired taste and is matched only by the attachment you have to circling a toilet bowl for hours on end. Demeaning is not quite the word I am looking for. More like a mission. So you plan your day and night like a military operation, because there is no room for play dates in the land of defaecograms.

Once your mission is accomplished, your bowel emptied and you feel like death, you wend your way to the hospital where they provide you with a cocktail that you are sure is more of a medical death wish. You are requested to sip this, but I am a lot smarter than that. I close my nose to avoid tasting the mixture, and within five minutes have passed the second test. Then they politely ask you to hang around for two hours. In retrospect, this is the time when you should go for the gap because what follows is quite indescribable.

---

10 A medication used to clean out the bowels prior to medical procedures

After two hours, you enter an x-ray room wearing a delightful surgical gown with a slit at the back. I know, you simply want to weep. Slowly from behind the curtain, they roll out what they affectionately refer to as their 'Ferrari'. It is like having an encounter with aliens. You simply cannot believe that this is happening to you, let alone that other people have survived the ordeal. Gingerly, you climb the stairs of the Ferrari. No, it does not feel like Everest in the least. Once on top, you look down on a commode. I kid you not. You sit down while two assistants stand by your side for reasons known only to them and G-d. Perhaps to prevent you from fleeing.

The radiologist seats himself in front of his equipment in his pristine, sealed-off section and instructions follow. I'll spare you further details, other than to say that the net result is to perform, as best you can, a bowel action. They do not particularly care how you do it, as long as you succeed. However, before you think this is an easy feat, there is more to this, so hold your breath. This performance is choreographed for prosperity in a video with your name and birthdate. Personally, I thought that this was the closest I would ever get to the Oscars. If they are not entirely happy with the results, you are swished off for an MRI, slid into a tunnel to listen to the latest drum solos from the cosmos. There are no words. When completed, you try your best to sit up, because by now your back is in spasm. You guessed correctly. Yes, your bowels are clear, but your back remains in spasm. You can't win all the wars.

And thus begins the dance of shame associated with pelvic floor. When your friends ask you what you did today, a live rendition of this journey would have them shaking their heads in disbelief and filling in forms for your admission to La La Land, as an involuntary patient for observation. So you keep quiet in total humiliation, and are not surprised that no self-respecting person who crosses your path has ever heard of the defaecogram trail, much less experienced it. Whatever follows this, in the form of vaginal and rectal examination, blood tests and pressure point release, can only be described as a walk in the park. They train you well.

Q Did you have any expectations regarding your first surgery?

The conclusion of the radiologist's report noted "the presence of a large enterocele[11] and a 6-cm diameter anterior rectocele which empties."

The nature of my first surgery in 2011 was a Pelvic Floor Reconstruction and Trans-Abdominal Repair using mesh. My anxiety related to the surgery was allayed by the fact that I had the best surgeon who was caring, receptive, respectful and compassionate. The quality of life prior to surgery, ravaged by pelvic organ prolapse and constant pain was a condition that I could not continue to live with. I believed that the surgery would be the catalyst for a different quality of life. I was also aware that my psychological welfare and support in this complex domain of surgery needed to be a parallel process. I did not view the surgeon as a cosmic teddy bear, the cure-all to ongoing symptomatology, whether it be physical, spiritual or psychological.

Some of my expectations were unrealistic. I anticipated being back at work within a month, with a new zest for life and the ability to navigate my daily life without constant, debilitating pain. I was aware that the operation would last many hours, requiring an intensity of focus and expertise. On the morning of the surgery, I met with both the anaesthetist and the colorectal surgeon, and was

11 A condition in which the small intestine moves down and press against the top part of the vagina

informed that the surgery would be abdominal in nature. I realised in a heartbeat that the sequel to surgery was not going to be a walk in the park.

Q At which point did you realise the enormity of the impact of the surgery?

I realised the enormity of the surgery on waking up in the Intensive Care Unit (ICU) on high doses of morphine to cope with the pain. But my thoughts were soon interrupted by a visit from a broad-smiling, highly charged and energetic presence in the form of a physiotherapist, or as I subsequently thought of him, a physio-terrorist. He looked like a man on a mission, determined to get me up and running, so to speak. But I could not run, walk, sit up or move on my own!

"Exercise is important if she wants to get strong, keep her moving," he told my then partner, a marathon runner and a participant in numerous Iron Man marathons, and at 69 still jogging his way around Johannesburg. He proceeded to lift my arms and with this movement came the realisation that my condition gave new meaning to the word vulnerable. Six hours of surgery, two days in ICU, and then on the road to recovery in the surgical ward. No sooner had they transferred me to my bed, surrounded by tubes, morphine pumps and the like, than my then partner whipped off my blankets and said, "Time to exercise. You heard what the physiotherapist said. Keep moving. Let's go for a walk."

In total disbelief, I whispered, "But I'm exhausted, have no strength and have only just been transferred from ICU!"

"My point exactly. I'm going to help you get strong again," he retorted.

Writhing in agony and doubled over, he tried to get me to stand up. "I can't do this," I said.

"Just around the nurse's station," he replied. I could not believe what was happening to me. I could barely get my legs off the bed and he had images of me walking around the nurse's station. I mean, around the whole of the nurses' station! It felt more like an invitation to climb Everest.

Thank G-d the matron walked past and upon seeing the look on my face, asked him, "What on earth are you doing?"

"Taking her for a brisk walk," he replied.

"You're not going anywhere," she retorted and blessedly tucked me back into bed.

The road to recovery from this point onwards would prove to be one of the most profound journeys of my life, unravelling and exposing deep wounds that had remained buried for years.

Q How did you cope following the surgery?

I coped well in the ward where I was for five days, receiving around-the-clock sound medical care. I did not cope very well at home.

I had to overcome the fear around moving and voiding post-surgery, navigating my world in this stitched-up, painful body. With the aid of Lyrica[12] anything is possible and in this state I dragged myself back to work six weeks later. In hindsight, I needed more time to recuperate, given the demands of the tender I was working on. I was told that I could work from home to accommodate my weakened state. Days and nights fused into one. I worked on a treadmill schedule. So I worked for a few hours

12 Schedule 6 painkillers

and then slept, then worked and then slept, on a twenty-four-hour cycle. By September 2012, the contract had come to an end. I had paid for it with my health.

In January 2013, fourteen months after my first surgery, I was referred for a second defaecogram and an MRI. The MRI findings noted a bilateral renal angle tenderness suggesting an underlying pyelonephritis[13]."

The colorectal surgeon referred me to the Pain Clinic. It was decided by the anaesthetist that to address the pain concerns, a Hypogastric Plexus and a Ganglion Impar Block[14] would be administered. This procedure was scheduled for the morning of 16 February 2013, four days prior to the second surgery. The initial block was the Ganglion Impar. Three minutes into this procedure, I had a general tonic-clonic seizure requiring a Cardiac Pulmonary Resuscitation (CPR).

My family was contacted and I remained in the hospital for 24 hours for observation. The pain in my chest from the CPR was intense, and the shock to me both physically and emotionally was immense. It caused much distress in the family system and brought us to the realisation that nothing could be taken for granted. I began to confront the possibility of a shortened life, and the myriad emotions and dialogues that surfaced around this notion.

In the end, the conclusion I reached was that it was the manner of my dying that concerned me more than death itself. I did not want my life to be a journey of ever-increasing disability, pain and suffering. I did not want to be a burden to my children. If it were not for my abiding faith in my surgeon and my Maker, I would

---

13 A severe kidney infection

14 A procedure performed to block nerve impulses in order to reduce chronic pelvic or rectal pain

never have contemplated surgery four days later. The months following the second surgery were more of the same.

Q **Did you return to work following the second surgery?**

My days were unpredictable, standing was difficult and I couldn't sit for any length of time because it would induce a pain cycle. An author/editor friend approached me to co-write a book, my focus being to explore the concept of suffering as it related to the Book of Job. This was the beginning of a journey into the metaphysical, meaning and faith, which served to comfort me through the years ahead. I had come to the realisation that a conventional eight-hour job was something that I could no longer manage. So it appeared as if the illness served as a catalyst for me to tap into other talents, which had remained dormant.

Q **How long were you well before you were facing another surgery?**

By December 2013, severe abdominal pain, bladder infections and Defaecation Obstructive Syndrome surfaced.

A CT scan revealed a deep-seated 2.7 x 2.6 collection in the pelvis to the left of the upper third of the rectum suggestive of diverticulitis[15]. There was also evidence of an umbilical hernia.

I consulted with the colorectal surgeon, who referred me to a physiotherapist for a six-month period of pressure point release and Biofeedback, following which my condition would be re-evaluated.

15 Inflammation of small, bulging pouches that can form in the lining of the digestive tract

We need normal tone and good muscle functioning to store and void food and water as they pass through the digestive system. Pressure point release is a type of massage that relieves muscular pain and readies the muscles for manipulation. Biofeedback equipment is used to measure conscious or unconscious body functioning, which is fed back in the form of visual or auditory signals. Patients are taught to use these signals to manipulate internal events that contribute to an illness. It can be used to increase activity in weak muscles or reduce spasms.

At the time I was on my fourth round of antibiotics for urinary infection with no positive results. I approached my gynaecologist, who upon doing both an anal and vaginal examination, as well as an ultrasound, detected a mass and referred me for an MRI. The results confirmed his suspicion and he referred me to the colorectal surgeon, who requested a second MRI.

Cautiously the surgeon suggested that he would only undertake a third surgery if he could enlist the team from the Pain Clinic, and consult with both my daughters prior to surgery.

The MRI findings were suggestive of complete pelvic floor failure.

Surgery found no bowel adhesions, the mesh was identified and removed, and replaced by Provine[16]. A pelvic cyst with a diameter of 50 x 5 cm was aspirated, removed and sent for histology. The pelvic organ prolapse was repaired. Findings of the biopsy revealed a Multicystic Peritoneal Mesothelioma condition associated with repeated pelvic surgeries.

In truth, I had viewed the third surgery as my last surgery, so it was planned to ensure an optimal outcome. It was a lengthy surgery with complications that set in in ICU. I was in hospital

16 A biological mesh

for a period of two and a half weeks, followed by admission to a step-down facility for an additional week. At my follow-up visit with the surgeon six weeks later, the surgery was declared a success.

But life is never that simple, is it? Seven months after the third surgery, I visited the gynaecologist, presenting with severe abdominal pain and resurfacing of the Defaecation Obstructive Syndrome. On clinical examination, it was evident that "the pubo-rectalis opening was constricted to such an extent as to preclude examination with a distal finger". In addition, I had a bladder infection, and on examination scar tissue was evident. I was subsequently referred to a Professor of Gynaecology who, following an examination, diagnosed a rectocele Grade III failure. This was corrected in a fourth surgery in June 2016.

At my follow-up visit the operation was declared a success. However, eight weeks later I became incontinent, requiring a fifth surgery to introduce a sling and a laparoscopy to examine the state of the internal organs.

Q How did you take control of managing your illness and your recovery?

I never settled for diagnoses that did not resonate with the subjective sense of what I was experiencing health-wise. If a diagnosis did not sit well with me, I dismissed it and searched for another opinion that did. This is your life that you are dealing with. To the doctor, you may just be another paying patient, but to you, your doctor is a significant person in the journey towards health. I am not sure specialists appreciate the importance of relationship in the prescription of health. It is far more than a placebo.

I remember when I was fighting for my life in ICU after my third abdominal surgery, when complications set in. I felt myself shifting between this world and another. In this haze, I looked up and the surgeon's eyes caught mine. He said, "You have to be strong now." And I understood. I had to be strong for both of us to pull through this ordeal. He needed my commitment to life, as much as I needed his skills to keep me from dying. It was about relationship, about reading the urgency in the subtext of his simple, short request, which went something like this: we both know you are in trouble here, and I am trying my very best. But I need your cooperation if both you and I are to survive this ordeal.

Q Was it difficult to make the shift from being healthy to being ill?

Any shift in personal identity demands the embracing of a new identity, and this is a process. When you lose a limb through trauma, the limb lives on in your consciousness, even though it is not physically there. The loss calls for a redefinition of self, from a person with full physical functioning to one who is now redefined as being disabled. This is a great wounding, and it takes time to adjust to the change in status, if you ever really do. So adaptation is not necessarily about reaching a destination; it is about accommodation, coupled with partial or real acceptance of what life has thrown at you at this particular stage of your life.

We all know people who use their illnesses to manipulate others. So instead of having an illness, they become the illness and use it as the primary currency of exchange. You can also prolong the illness longer than is necessary, or stall achieving those things you want for your life. I often wondered whether I was using my illness to hide from responsibilities that I may have wanted to avoid. However, over time I reconciled myself with the fact that this was not so, but it took a lot of soul searching.

In retrospect, so much was accomplished, requiring so many shifts, at a time of life when one should have more freedom. Jung proposed that in the first half of life women focus mainly on their family and those persons in their inner circle of care. This is her prime responsibility, while her husband navigates the external world of career, finance and family security. Women's prowess has, for the most part, been defined by their cultural contexts, values and belief systems.

Times have changed. By the second half of life, a woman's ambit of interaction with the external world shifts. No longer is she preoccupied with raising children. For many, there has been a gradual acceptance of their bodily changes over time, especially after menopause. Many women at this stage of life are savouring the freedom to choose a life they may have put on hold for many years. With children leaving home, new interests develop, couples face new ways of connecting with each other or separating paths. There is also the freedom that comes with unprotected intercourse without fear of pregnancy.

Q What was the resultant impact of prolonged illness and repeated surgeries?

Each surgery took me to the depths of despair, to the edge of the abyss with an unrelenting force. Although faith felt etched into my very being, it did not manage to quell the pain that scratched though my body. It would prove to be one of the most profound journeys that I had ever undertaken, unravelling and exposing deep wounds that had remained buried for years. The wars not won, the battles not fought, the loves not surviving because they were unbalanced and the journey not taken for fear that the spirit was too weak.

It was the catalyst for my journey into exploring illness as metaphor.

- » Why pelvic floor?
- » Why me?
- » Why now?
- » If symptoms and illness represent the soul's suffering, then what was the suffering symbolic of?
- » What could remedy this suffering, and where and how would it find a voice?
- » Does suffering find us, or do we find suffering?

The questions were relentless, but the exploration of them proved to be profound.

I do not believe that we are wired for certain illnesses. Rather, I believe we have a propensity for an illness given our genetic makeup, and then in conjunction with our environment and lived experience, we develop a tendency towards presenting with symptoms which, if unaddressed on a psychological or spiritual level, result in illness. The journey served as a catalyst for the peeling away of my history, which lay etched in my biology. And with the unpeeling and confrontation of the wounding, a range of emotions surfaced.

To be struck down with illness on the cusp of a new life can be devastating, as this was not part of the master plan. When a symptom evolves into chronic illness and a compromised quality of life long term, the effects are challenging for both the women and their partners.

There is much grief during this period and usually very little support. Life carries on, as do the commitments we have. And as the months and years march on, so do the financial implications of the illness. I kept thinking, "There has to be a superior replacement to all of this." But what would it be, and what form would it take? It was no ordinary audit of financial accountability. It was an audit of the costs of the illness, and there were many.

Illness also heralds a life stage in which there is an altered and often drastic reduction in the active lives of patients, resulting in increased compromise in social roles. The sick role knocks at the door, causing a biographical rupture that signals the onset of body failure and its resultant consequences encompass many losses. The patient comes under the scrutiny of all systems as the roles change and adaptations to the illness set in. No facet of one's life remains untouched, bringing with it a renewed sense of vulnerability. While not life-threatening, the symptoms I experienced did impact negatively on my quality of life and sense of wellbeing. Psychologically, I experienced symptoms of depression, anxiety, fatigue and the inevitable side-effects of the various pain medications.

Q Where did you find comfort during this difficult time, and what insights did you glean that were helpful along the way?

I never felt abandoned. I confronted my need for spirituality, which could only accurately be described as a deep and abiding hunger of the soul. I realised that healing is a complex phenomenon, requiring me to reintegrate the fragments of the life I once knew, before the onset of chronic illness. I saw it as my calling, and it did serve as the catalyst for the exploration for the meaning of my life.

You can die of your illness and be healed. Your body can be ravaged by illness and your soul can be healed. It depends on your worldview and perspective. I began to appreciate every nuance of health and it most certainly taught me to live in the moment with immense gratitude. So many people die in an instant, without warning, without preparation. I chose to soldier on despite the struggle, to take back what could be retrieved. I fought for the quality that I believed was mine and tried to rekindle a belief in a tomorrow.

Q How did you make sense of your illness and the suffering that it brought?

I familiarised myself with various models of illness, in a quest to understand more of the mind-body connection. I have a Clinical Masters in Social Work, a background in Reiki and am familiar with the chakra system and the impact that psychological wounding has on the mind-body connection. My growing awareness of the energy systems of the body and their role in diagnostics and healing aided my understanding of illness and healing.

At the outset of my journey, the presenting problem of chronic pain and compromised body functioning were the sole focus of my required intervention. The symptoms were equated with dysfunction in the bodily system, and the natural assumption I made was that once surgery repaired the cause of the symptoms, functionality would return and my life would return to normal. Over time, I became increasingly aware of the enormity of the needs of patients on all fronts that were necessary for optimal healing.

I say this with the utmost humility. I had the best surgeons, who were caring, receptive, respectful and compassionate. But the healing of the body was not a parallel process to the healing of the psyche.

Surgeons live highly charged lives, their work fraught with intricacies within the human body. Their operations last many hours and the intensity of focus required is considerable. All their expertise comes into play when they walk beside you into theatre.

Psychological support in the complex domain of pelvic floor surgery needs to be a parallel process, whether it comes in the form of individual and/or couple intervention or support groups. It takes a remarkably resilient, compassionate and strong presence to deal with the onslaught of post-operative adjustments and to handle them with the maturity and integrity that the patient and her partner may require.

Referring patients to psychiatrists because their symptoms do not fit an existing diagnosis further labels patients who often feel a deep sense of shame around this very issue. Dismissing a patient when a doctor cannot make sense of the symptoms is not the logical step in the continuum of care. When you are suffering and surgeons have little more to offer or are unable to make sense of the suffering in physical terms, you slowly, but surely begin to feel that the subtext reads something like this: "You know, other patients do not react this way. Maybe there is a psychological component here."

But then I began to explore the research and this attitude was negated by the research findings. The more I read, the more I realised that there were no real cures for pelvic floor disorder, merely temporary interventions that required more surgery if and when they failed.

It was a journey, not a one-stop repair. And many women with whom I spoke afterwards had similar tales to tell.

According to Kurts Strange, the direct result of medical specialisation is the isolation, ignoring for the most part the mind-body connection. Treatment is therefore one-dimensional. In addition, the medical model has failed to accept the extent to which healing requires relationships which will lead to trust, hope, and a sense of wellbeing for patients. Failure to recognise this is costly to patients, systems, and entire communities. Returning to a state of well-being incorporates shifts in mind, body and spirit, ensuring an improvement in the quality of life for the patient, both prior to and during a medical intervention. Health is not the absence of disease. Health is far more than this.

Q Were there any particular models of illness that you resonated with?

I began to explore various health models. The Health within Illness Model (HWIM) highlights the polarity of health and illness that coexist in the existential realities of people living with chronic illness. The premise of the model is that health is not linear and that the self in experience of illness is in constant motion. The individual's body is viewed as being-in-the-world and the self is viewed as personal identity, a conscious being sharing the world with others. The model views illness as a life course derailed by losses, which disconnects the unity between body and self, and self and the world.

Suffering is experienced as inner turmoil that is not given a voice and shared with others. The more we suffer, the more likely we are to present with a symptom or illness. Our inner suffering is therefore presented to the world as a metaphor. In chronic disease, suffering would be directly correlated with a sense of helplessness and hopelessness. Chronic illness is the catalyst for exposing suffering brought on by unexplored losses and anger, restricting the patient's power to exist.

Patients need to respect themselves, to listen to their symptoms, to respect their limits and pace themselves. Within the constraints of illness, they need to regain power over their lives. Suffering is the catalyst that forces the sufferer to change their perspectives on life, the world, their relationships and their health. It also challenges them to view time differently, grabbing the fleeting well-moments, opening their hearts to explore a spiritual journey, reinvesting in their lives and owning their life story.

I viewed my own suffering as the catalyst for my growth, a challenge to search for and re-evaluate the meaning of my life. I am convinced that had I not done this, I would have been left with the hollow experience of existential emptiness and despair. I needed to and did grapple with the essence of who I was, sans accomplishments. In other words, who had I become as soul during this lifetime?

I may have appeared fragile, but on the inside I felt like an awakening giant. What I had thought was important in years past, now seemed to be of little value. I gained clarity through journaling about journeys, past and present, noticing lessons learnt, pervading themes and tried to make sense of the fragmentation that I was confronting. It provided me with a depth of understanding, and a realisation that while G-d's framework is divine, man is limited by his human understanding. It forced me to confront my frailty and my strengths, and served as a catalyst for living my ordinary life in an extraordinary way. It called for an integration of my lived experience and my life's purpose, against the backdrop of my own human limitations, within the context of the life I had lived. I began to realise that even though my body was failing me, it did not detract from me and my worth. They were two different processes. I never felt flawed because of the illness. Rather the illness was the catalyst to explore the avenues that were flawed.

CHAPTER TWO

PAIN

I have included my diary extract on pain to highlight the various meanings it had for me, the areas it forced me to address and the role it played in my citizenship in the land of the ill. There is physical pain, emotional pain and spiritual pain, and on some level, they became entwined in my narrative and healing. So I shall share these with you and begin by reflecting on the gift of pain, as I now see it.

The cleanser called pain

On a purely physical level, pain is a form of suffering, but it is a masterful teacher. The pain that we walk with on the inside is not tangible or visible to the outside world. It is a quiet, inner, often desperate scream to be acknowledged, attended to and comforted.

Without coming to terms with the anguish surrounding pain, we are unable to walk forward. So in a sense, it brings us to our knees and keeps us there, forcing us to lift our heads and look forward. But we need acceptance of the pain, and to understand its meaning and why it grinds away at us, day in and day out. And if the pain lingers particularly long, then I see it as an incapacity brought on by the Divine to stop us in our tracks and take stock. This is one aspect. In taking stock, we need to be able to analyse the costs, own them and be able to put them someplace comfortable within our being. I used pain in a transformative sense, as is the case in writing this book.

Personal pain and physical pain can often be associated with loss. When we wake up to loss and address it, it becomes an invitation to look at our suffering with more compassion for ourselves. We might identify the loss, but not be able to process it. However, the integration of the two is essential to its resolution. For me, pain was the signifier of the lessons not learnt, the paths not taken. What it brought in its wake restored my sense of worth and made the suffering that much more meaningful. Those long, dark hours, those years of suffering forced me to deal with these aspects through prayer, journaling, contemplation and therapy. I searched every corner, explored every crevice, learnt patience, endurance, humility and sacrifice.

Pain brought isolation, loneliness and aloneness – all the gifts the prophets sought when they left the mainstream and travelled up the mountains and into the caves to explore the darkness within. And when the exploration was done, the healing completed, they emerged again, to face anew the journey, ready to teach and transform. For it is in the cave, the shadow, the unconscious, the dark crevices of our being, that the gold is to be found. Pain's isolation broadened my depth of understanding of myself and there was a direct correlation between the pain and my connection to G-d.

Pain my healer

Pain was the signal to start the healing journey that I was always meant to take. I began to question everything in earnest. Sometimes I found answers; other times I realised that I didn't need to know the answer. What I needed to learn was to ask the right questions and then live the answers that came to me through the breeze in short staccato sound bites. Sometimes there was a crescendo of insight; at others, a diminuendo, but truth be told, when they balanced out, I was still one step ahead on the journey. It was the crescendos and diminuendos that allowed me to catch my breath, as the pain subsided or began to escalate.

It taught me detachment from the small things in life that others thought were monumental. It taught me about the essential, that more was not better and less not something diminished. It also highlighted the areas of my life where I had been wounded and where healing was needed.

And ultimately, it taught me that without the grace of G-d, healing would never take place. That even in death, healing can take place, because it is not measured in earthly terms.

It is the healing of the psyche and the soul, of the unfinished journey, of mastery of the grand plan and my own unique ground plan being resolutely served to the finish line.

Pain my protector

More than anything else throughout this entire journey, of one thing I could be certain, and that was that Pain would accompany me every day. It became my companion. It signalled me and guided me when it thought that I was doing too much. It flared up like a temper when it felt that I was letting symptoms linger too long and required that they be attended to. Pain forced me to stand still, to listen to my inner landscape until I could no longer bear the screams and had to look for a healer, one who would listen without judgement.

Pain brought me to my knees, but taught me so much. It taught me to honour the symptoms of my body; when to withdraw from the pulse of life and when to venture into the world. It immobilised me when I thought that I was ready to run. It kept me at home, protected and alone, and in this state the rumblings started. It started like a thief in the night, a tiny tap, a whisper. It would wake me deep in the night with words tumbling into my conscious mind. I would wake up knowing that this was the moment that needed to be written about. And what came forth had little to do with ranting and raving against the pain and against the moon. It had to do with the unconscious awakening and demanding to be explored, to be analysed, and ultimately to be shared with others.

This was going to be an unusual tale in its delivery. How else does one talk about the obvious and reflect its magnitude and debilitating features as it seeps into every crevice of your being, every joint, every muscle, every memory that holds it captive and every desire that must be freed. And so, in time, the journaling resulted as a response to the pain. It gave it a voice in a way that was not painful.

But as time wore on it served to discern where I would go, how long I could stay, when the exit bell would ring and when it was time to go home and pop another pain killer for a few hours of relief. It had no hour; it had no preference for the season; it often did not have a preferred point of attack, but the inflammation that caused it told a story. Of a mind scorched with painful memories, of unexpressed traumas, of cruelty and of betrayal, rejection and shame. All these were embedded in this body of mine, stored up, waiting to be released and to be shared with others in a way they could relate to.

And so I began to play with my friend and see how much pain I could tolerate. I tried to outsmart it, but it taught me its lesson well. I learnt to catch it at the first sensation and that initial glimpse taught me to go for chemical cover. This nipped the onslaught in the bud, and taught me that I could be an equal player and control the game of pain. It made me live in awe of the human condition, the human body and its resilience to soldier on. It made me view others with compassion. It taught me how easily and relentlessly we judge without empathy, understanding or compassion, never knowing what sapped others of their energy. This ravaging friend called Pain taught me to be strong and stoic, to complain little and to soldier on despite.

Q What is the requirement for the diagnosis of pain from a medical perspective?

To qualify for the diagnosis, pain must have been continuous or recurrent for a minimum period of six months. In addition, the presence of an underlying infection or obvious pathology must be excluded. Pain is often assumed to be caused by either organic or psychological factors, but not both. Psychological factors are usually attributed to pain when physical underpinnings cannot be located.

Chronic pelvic pain (CPP) presents a major challenge to healthcare professionals owing to its complex aetiology[17] and poor response to therapy. It is defined as chronic or persistent pain perceived in structures related to the pelvis of either men or women. It is often associated with negative cognitive, behavioural, sexual and emotional consequences as well as with symptoms suggestive of lower urinary tract, sexual, bowel, pelvic floor or gynaecological dysfunction. Generally, chronic pain leads to avoidance, thus the importance of reversing the cycle. Acute pain is known to affect mood, memory, attention, thoughts and behaviour, and impacts on the central nervous system.

---

17 The cause(s) of a disease or condition

The development of healthy coping strategies is essential to avoiding the downward spiral that pain has on the functioning of the individual's daily functioning. Patients need to be educated about the impact pain has on their lives, and be given assistance with pain management. Many women who have undergone pelvic floor surgery present with chronic pelvic pain, negative psychological, behavioural and sexual consequences, sexual dysfunction, anger, frustration and depression, all of which directly impact on relationship satisfaction.

Kaplan et al (2014) argue that depression, chronic anxiety and PTSD are neuro-inflammatory and neuro-degenerative conditions, which left untreated lead to disability and incapacity. He views depression and pain as extreme outlets for microglial[18] inflammation, which reignites pain and compromises the individual's ability to heal. His strategy is to treat the whole person, not the symptom.

It is thought that patients who present with chronic pain invariably present with a history of emotional, physical and infectious assaults. Unlike acute pain, chronic pain appears to cause chemical signalling to change in the nervous system. Long-term use of analgesics, sedatives and drugs often leads to stomach problems, lethargy and constipation, and reduced activity often results in physical deterioration. Little wonder that patients often experience excessive suffering and disability.

Programmes to address chronic pain set out to determine the nature of the patient's pain, its treatable cause, and whether pain is acute or chronic in nature. Treatment options are then explored with the patient, the goals they set out for themselves in terms of

18 Cells located throughout the brain and spinal cord that are the first line of immune defence in the central nervous system

pain management as well as any obstacles that exist and how they will be dealt with.

Off the beaten track

During the course of my illness the narrative of pain has surfaced in different ways. The post-operative pain was understandable. However, I expected it to be of limited duration, diminishing in intensity as recuperation progressed. Chronic pain is more debilitating because it is ongoing, incapacitating, affecting every aspect of your life: mood, mobility, resilience, social contact and overall sense of well-being. It was during this period that I was prescribed opiates for pain control. Opiate side effects simply compounded the quality-of-life issues I confronted, and over time the opiates became less effective, requiring more frequent administration.

During this period, a close friend was working with a client who had commissioned the writing of a spiritual trilogy. He shared with my friend that in addition to being a chartered accountant, he had been gifted with healing abilities since childhood and was a devout Christian. He asked her whether there was any particular area of her life that she needed to heal. In response, she told him about my ongoing condition and requested healing from him on my behalf. Unbeknown to me, he agreed to intercede and the following morning he sent her an email to say that the request for healing had been granted by G-d and the Christ. In the email, he noted that in five days the core issues would be attended to and healing would occur during the following five days.

Knowing how sceptical I was about things of this nature, my friend did not share this information with me. The telephonic contact had taken place on 11 April 2014. Healing would be completed by 21 April 2014. In the email, he cautioned that I needed to be weaned off the opiates as these were adversely affecting my health.

At the time, when I woke up in the mornings it was difficult to move my body, as each movement seemed to induce more pain. So I would hold onto the slats of my headboard and manoeuvre my body ever so slowly to accommodate the pain until I lay on my left side. From this angle, using the Alexander technique, I would attempt a sitting position. Once seated, I would gingerly attempt to stand, and when confident that I was stable, venture to walk. It would take a while before I could walk around with ease. Generally, I would make my way to the kitchen, make myself a cup of tea and then seat myself in the lounge where a medical heating pad awaited me to ease the pain and discomfort.

Unaware of the contract between my friend and the healer, my life continued as 'normal'. On 21 April 2014, I awoke to find myself turning onto my left side. As this happened, the strangeness of this movement confused me. I had not experienced any pain. The debilitating nerve pain that had gripped me each day was not present on this day. I cautiously sat up, then stood up with ease and without any leg pain, and made my way to the kitchen in what seemed like an altered state.

I was totally confused by this turn of events. I made myself a cup of tea and went to sit in the lounge. There I sat for two hours, waiting for the pain to return. But nothing changed. In total confusion I phoned my friend and told her what had transpired. She laughed and asked me to go to my computer and open an email she was about to send me. I did as instructed and read the email the healer had sent her two weeks prior.

"You need to phone and thank him," she suggested. But I did not do this because while intellectually I was confronted with what seemed to me an inexplicable flight into health, I certainly did not trust the process. So I waited patiently for the bubble to burst and the pain to return, but this did not happen. Ten days later I phoned to thank him for the healing. He corrected me, saying that he was merely the conduit, that the healing had been given by G-d. He also urged me to contact the doctors to wean me off the opiates.

You can imagine the medical fraternity's response to my request to be weaned off opiates. I was well aware that they must have thought that my judgement was compromised or that I had totally lost the plot. It took three weeks before they agreed to wean me off opiates, under the supervision of the psychiatrist attached to the Pain Clinic.

The morning of admission arrived and the psychiatrist met with me to explain the possible risks involved in opiate withdrawal. I listened intently. Then he explained that back-up medication for pain would be made available. I told him that I wanted no additional drugs to be prescribed at that time. I explained that it was important for me to reach baseline functioning in order to ascertain how I would cope without any chemical intervention. He seemed rather concerned at my stance.

I explained to him what had transpired with the healer, showed him the emails confirming the interchange and he agreed to respect my wishes. Other than increased anxiety and kaleidoscopic experiences during the withdrawal stage, the opiate withdrawal ran smoothly and once weaned, I experienced no pain.

I returned home without chemical backup for pain. What I did require was medication for sleep disturbance, apparently one of the side effects of opiate withdrawal.

Since that withdrawal from opiates I have experienced post-surgical, breakthrough pain and pain associated with evacuation. But the intensity of pain that warranted opiates has never returned.

Q How did you learn to cope with the illness over time?

The mourning of the slow onset of many losses over a six-year period brought with it, no, more to the point, demanded that I live despite the pain.

When I asked, "Why me?" the answer was silence.

When I asked, "Why now?" there was silence.

When I asked, "When will the healing come, if ever?" the answer from the void, was silence.

When I asked, "When will I live without pain?" Not a squeak.

When I asked, "For how much longer?" Nothing.

When I asked whether it was worth carrying on, my soul said, "Yes!"

There were no avenues for sharing this grief, no fellow storytellers, no shared comfort. So the grief for me was ongoing, a response to all the small losses along the way. Transforming the struggle, bitterness, anger, depression and grief by committing to writing this book brought meaning to my life. Transforming the loss and making the best of it, I rebuilt my sense of self, but it took time. I learned to live with loss and dance to its rhythm.

The gift of loneliness ignited my soul's longing to give voice to the journey. What a gift this was for me, to be alone and lonely and to sit quietly exploring the answers, to savour the journey. People would rather be shredded than be left alone, such is their fear of it. They will stay in marriages of quiet desperation and abuse, rather than leave and be alone. They would rather put up with virtually anything and pay the psychic price, than be alone. As you attune to the inner and outer landscapes, as you review and reflect, loneliness can be transformed into a spiritually charged journey.

When you realise that no one notices the hand grasping for connection, that no one answers the call of despair, loneliness can tear away at our being. Isolation and loneliness are an invitation to exist in a meaningful field of experience. They confront our deepest needs for belonging, acceptance, validation and closeness. It is the experience that connects us to others, that makes us realise that no man is an island. It is the catalyst for self-awareness, and often the catalyst for going in search of community and belonging. I was one of the lucky ones. I held on like a rabid dog until I could find a way to transform the feeling of the void and emptiness.

The birth of a new relationship with myself made it all worth it in the end. We need to be able to sit with our own pain and the pain of others, wait for it to subside, and recommit to life. To be able to live through the anguished nights of pain, both physical and emotional, and soldier on nonetheless, takes great courage.

CHAPTER THREE

LOSS

In time I became deeply and irrationally resentful that the dreams I had for the second half of my life were being deleted in the wink of an eye. I was angry that there was no one to turn to in this vulnerable state. I watched the life I had known run like mercury through my fingers. I had forgotten who I was or what health felt like. There was the lingering fear that maybe this would never go away.

Looking through the barbed wire fence from the side of illness, I glimpsed some of the many losses over time. By far the most important loss was the loss of certainty. And with the loss of certainty came the realisation that:

» Illness has brought with it a feeling of energy leakage symbolic of the onset of body failure.
» Illness began to represent my dance with health, life and death.
» Illness heralded a life stage characterised by a drastic reduction in activity and compromised social roles.
» Illness demanded changes in schedules, doctor's visits and rehabilitation and relapses.

- » Illness replaced my former sense of cohesion only to be replaced by a sense of chaos.
- » Illness equalled a renewed sense of vulnerability and mortality.
- » Illness made it difficult to return to a normal life and begin again.
- » Illness demanded that I live in a new way.
- » Illness taught me that patients need to take control of their own recovery as far as possible.
- » Illness taught me about the need to be resilient.
- » Illness forced me to turn to myself, others and the Divine because we are all connected and responsible for each other.

SOME OF THE MANY LOSSES

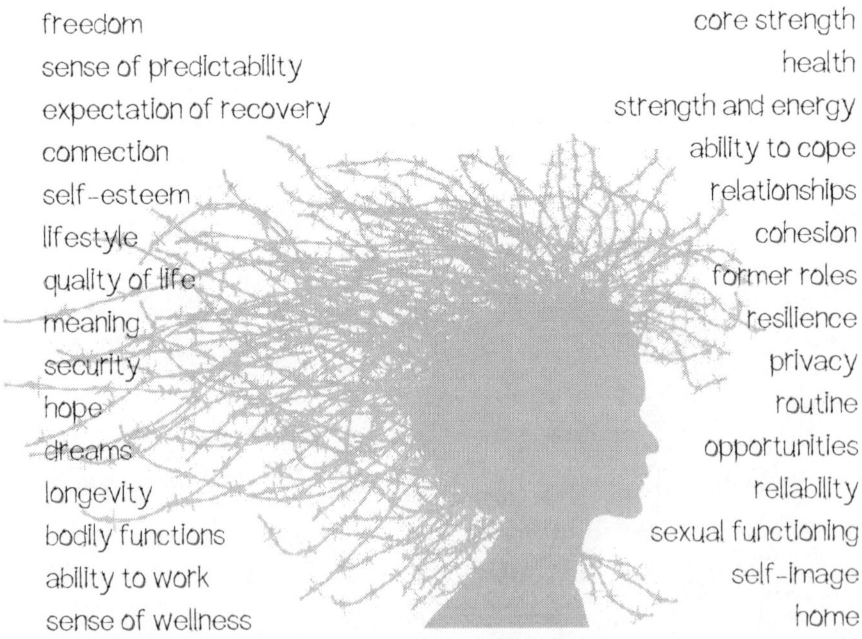

Unspoken systemic losses

Shortly after my second surgery, my elder brother, approaching his 70th birthday, started losing weight. He would stand in front of me showing me how he could now wear trousers he had not worn in years. But then something strange happened. He stopped dieting, but continued to lose weight. His trim body became frail, and he gradually lost his ability to swallow. Nutrition took the form of sucking on fizz pops because they were easy to digest. Medical tests came back negative. He had also developed partial paralysis in his right leg, which hindered his ability to walk.

In my own post-surgery state, I became increasingly fearful that I was on a downward spiral to nowhere. It was then that the telephone rang. It was my brother informing me that he had been diagnosed with Stage 4 cancer of the stomach and oesophagus, and had a year to live. I was in total shock. In that split-second I committed to be there for him until his death.

This incident was the last straw in what was beginning to feel like a litany of losses, and resulted in my official dance with depression.

Ten years prior I had relocated to Johannesburg, following the death of my brother's daughter in the tsunami in Thailand. When I saw him again, a week after he told me his diagnosis and prognosis, I knew that he would not be celebrating his 70th birthday. I decided that I would be there for him. I found any excuse to contact him during the day, as I watched him stare out of the window waiting for the grim reaper.

At the time, I was involved with a man, an angry man, a man fraught with pain. He had a 15-year-old son who suffered from

Canavan disease[19], who lived with him at home. His son was bedbound, blind, physically and mentally challenged, tube-fed, mute and an angel. When you walked into his room, an air of grace, of pure undiluted essence greeted you. I watched as his father cared, shared, nurtured and loved him, this fragile soul who had been placed in his care. His son was his life, his purpose. Without his son, he couldn't navigate this world. His son was the source of his identity, his worth, his dignity, his compassion, his endurance, his love and his commitment.

His son's death was a slow, arduous death over the next three years. I felt like I was living with the survivor of some terrible atrocity. His son flourished through all this, because he had a father like no other. But in this dedication, there was little space for connection with me, his partner. His son and I were the two people that he cared for with a devotion I had never experienced. As my illness set in, his son's health began to decline, and everything changed.

Then his son died. In fact, there were so many deaths. He had lost a daughter, a son, a business, the very meaning of his life. I was aware that he cared for me deeply, but we were both deeply unhappy, and our relationship had a great deal to do with that. I realised far too late that I had entered a relationship based on my deep need not to be abandoned and to be taken care of.

But a wounded animal cannot flee. Instead, I did what I had done all my life when the odds seemed insurmountable. I withdrew and became silent. I felt like a captive of my own making. I was ill, not able to work and not in possession of the psychic strength required to leave and start again. I began to confront the painful

---

19 A rare, inherited degenerative disorder that damages the nerve cells in the brain so that they cannot send and receive messages

phenomenon of leaving. I lingered in a portal of discontent, a no man's land where alienation is marked, and emotional survival hangs on a thread. The fear of not coping was so overwhelming that I remained hostage to a conflictual context that scarred my soul. The emotional journey is compounded by fear and the realisation that healing takes a very long time, if it happens at all. A relationship was ending at the same time as I was facing losses on a multitude of levels. I left after my second surgery.

Q What has been the trajectory of your illness, its systemic losses and adaptation required over time?

The trajectory of the journey is often not spoken about. The silence is partly a collusion between the patient, the family system, and the medical fraternity. It encompasses the unspoken fears and hopes silenced by the various players because none are able to find within themselves the wherewithal to speak, hear or cope with the truth of their hopes and fears. There is no room for evaluation, transparency, dialogues that seek an alternative narrative. There is no time or willingness for all of this.

Q So what happens to all the unspoken aspects surrounding pelvic floor intervention, the high road and the low road?

The health of any given system is determined by the number of unspoken truths that are denied a voice. Like secrets, these unspoken truths, whether they exist in our personal lives, our marriages, our families, our communities or the medical fraternity treating our condition, have a life force of their own and become more and more difficult to avoid.

This book is an attempt to look truth in the eye. To those surgeons and specialists who crossed my path who were not only willing, but truthful in their understanding of the possible road ahead, I need to thank you for the forthrightness and bravery it took to talk about the difficulties inherent in the journey. Few understand the enormous responsibility that surgeons take upon themselves when they enter into a contract with you to do the best they can with what they have in the interest of your health. I am acutely aware that many of them are sometimes left feeling like they may have failed the patient nonetheless, as the fallout of the surgery does not reflect the intended outcome. But know that I do not sit in judgement of this because the intricacies of the task at hand and the willingness to partner me on this journey were taken upon jointly, with both parties profoundly aware of the costs inherent in the outcome.

I was forced to evaluate and confront the many unspoken truths associated with pelvic floor prolapse. I have tried to talk about them in such a way as to invite others to begin to voice those inherent in their personal journey – in a way that brings openness, acceptance and the capacity to give a voice to the difficult truths that have accompanied them on this particular journey into health.

The challenge following any diagnosis is to learn to live with the illness, adapting to the many challenges along the way. I view the adaptations within two categories: short-term adaptations and long-term adaptations. The shift between the two can often prove to be quite challenging, if not overwhelming. Most of us who become ill expect a period of compromised mobility, followed by a return to the nearest approximation of our lives prior to the onset of illness. Others are graced with a quality of life superior to the one prior to the onset of illness. But when the realisation sets in that the condition will be life-long, the impact can be overwhelming.

The quality-of-life shifts, the coping skills and resilience it demands of us are often more than we bargained for. The challenge is to facilitate the adaptation and hopefully rein in the demands of the illness rather than letting the illness rein in the quality of our lives. I was sufficiently mature to realise that this journey towards health would encompass a period of time. I never expected my life to return to the quality of life pre-surgery, but did envisage a level of health that would enhance my daily quality of life.

However, by the time I had reached the six-year mark, I realised that the initial onset and slow progression of my illness had reached a point where it would accompany me in the foreseeable future. It had become a chronic condition, presenting with ongoing knock-on effects that I was unable to field.

My perspectives changed, allowing me to dispassionately view the costs of the illness in the cold light of day. And the costs seem to have won in the end, especially the financial ones.

The cost of medical specialisation made me realise that in essence it is true that the patient is the one whose interests are lost in a system without interdisciplinary accountability for referral, updating colleagues on findings, etcetera. Each specialisation focuses on an area of the body with its associated symptomology. This constricted and limited viewpoint loses sight of the fact that the specialist is not dealing with a symptom, he is dealing with a human being who presented with a symptom. This keyhole vision negates the presence of a human being comprising an integrated system of body parts functioning simultaneously.

Medical personnel should be aware of the long-term financial implications of illness. Ongoing supportive interventions allow for the diminishing likelihood of prolapse recurring. Compliance with treatments ensure optimal outcome of surgeries.

As financial costs escalate, fewer and fewer funds are available to ensure that the patient can have a better quality of life. When the individual has to choose between healthcare and daily necessities for living, they are essentially faced with a Hobson's choice. It stands to reason then that financial constraints impact on the management requirements and plans of the individual.

As illness intrudes into every corner of one's life, there is a direct impact on one's mental health, brought in large part by the isolation that illness brings in its wake for patients long term. Over time, the financial costs of the illness preclude the individuals from attending to other aspects of their lives requiring budgetary discretion.

Long-term loss associated with chronic illness

Symptoms of prolapse are prolapse-specific. Over a six-year period one develops a keen sensitivity to the inner landscape of one's body and the symptoms that arise over time. These warning symptoms alert one to the changes inherent in the narrative of prolapse failure and recurrence over time. Each kind of prolapse confronted me with different symptomatology resulting in a different impact and requiring a different response both pre- and post-surgery.

By the six-year mark, I realised that the disruption of the illness would always partner me in a systemic dance of body failure. With the knock-on effect comes the realisation that the body is less resilient, as are you as a function of aging. You do not bounce back so quickly because of the toll exacted by ongoing surgery-and-recovery. Over time the illness disruption introduces a new concept of biographical time, signalled by the body's increasing default to failure and it resultant consequences.

The chaos is both internal and external and can prove to be most challenging. But as time ticks by, you realise that the life you had known has changed forever and that there will be no revisiting your former self. As you cope with ongoing demands and challenges, you are also confronted with uncertainty, new fears, unrecognised new symptoms demanding adaptability and fortitude over time. Aging brings with it compromised functioning in many areas, but when illness is a parallel process, the decline is more marked, forcing one to confront the cost of the journey head on.

Systemic role changes and costs

Family members bear witness to the narrative of illness from its initial diagnosis, through surgery followed by recovery, each stage presenting different emotional and physical challenges. You notice how family members start to keep a close eye on you, looking for clues that will alert them to any changes, however subtle. They become observers of a script that unfolds, a script that they are called upon to be involved with in various ways. And gradually, roles, tasks and priorities are reorganised, especially around the role of mother in the family.

I believe that these shifts force the next generation to confront their own aging and possibly their own mortality. To the family system as a whole, it brings to mind the meaning of health and illness and sometimes death. There were many deaths of family members and friends that took place over the course of those six years which highlighted the transitory nature of life. Nothing was taken for granted and life began to be lived with a renewed sense of appreciation.

The passage of life became a reality for all and the possibility of death, such a natural process in any small community in days gone by, was a re-emerging gift at this time. It was rich, it was real and it was human, and none of us avoided conversations we needed to have. It was not morbid because the discussions were paramount in raising interesting existential questions concerning the meaning of life as well as death, and mostly the brevity of it all. I think each person in the system did their own soul searching. It was a growth experience for all concerned.

The regressions that accompanied my illness, especially post-surgery, demanded role shifts. I remember when I had to resort to wearing nappies after my first operation. I had run out of the nappies that look like panties and the pharmacists only had the ones available where you stick down the sides. Obviously, I was unable to put them on by myself. So my daughter had to put a nappy on me while my granddaughter looked on. I made fun of it and we laughed till we cried, but it was not a laughing matter in terms of the meaning it held for all of us.

The role reversal of caring for a mother was a reality that surfaced time and time again over the years, more markedly after each surgery. My children took great strain during this period, depending on my response to each surgery. The CPR was a cataclysmic event for all of us and forced everyone to confront the possibility of a shortened life.

My role in relationship to my children became more limited. One of my daughters commented prior to my third surgery: "I am not ready for you to die. Who will mentor me going forward? Who will mentor me spiritually? Who will I be able to ask for guidance?" These questions were affirming for me because they spoke to a relationship of substance. But I knew that the impact of my death would be significant for many within the system, children and grandchildren aside. My children and grandchildren are experiencing the same gift I had when my father was ill over a lengthy period of time, but with one significant difference. We can dialogue our fears and the outcome. With my father, who suffered from Parkinson's disease, speech was not possible and therefore there was no medium to share our hopes, dreams and grief. When bonds are strong and discourse is open, the period of illness can be an enriching time for everyone. It provides an opportunity to speak the unspoken and attend to the unfinished conversations, and the healing this brings.

Progressive illness brings home that time marches on, that roles change and the systems cope better if they are cohesive. It is a challenging, exhausting and enriching experience. Much support is needed for those in the system whose lives are affected, whether this be children, spouses or friends. And a supportive structure is advised during this period as the changes force confrontations with new realities, fears and hopes.

So yes, while the illness happened in present time, it was the catalyst for conversations that surfaced about past and future, and it was these very conversations that highlighted the adaptations and coping skills that were needed going forward, as were new solutions to ongoing symptoms as they arose.

So illness heralded the beginning of the writing of a new chapter, of a new life reflection, new limitations, new adjustments, new conversations and a revised narration of the illness and its impact. It goes without saying that the emotional roller coaster is taxing for all concerned. The loss of aspects of self and the redefinition of self is a complex patchwork of the new social roles.

CHAPTER FOUR

ILLNESS AS METAPHOR – A CASE STUDY IN SHAME

> *The power of the clergy has waned and been supplanted by a new priest, in a white coat instead of black. Frans Kafka warns us not to place our faith in the external quantifiable world reflective of the twentieth century. He holds that our wounds are to the soul, and only that which reaches the soul can bring about healing. The physician is seen as the servant of nature. The physician does not heal; nature heals.*
>
> *When the body is broken the physician may promote conditions that facilitate healing, but he cannot heal the wounds to the soul. Decades ago D.H. Lawrence realised this:*
>
> *"I am not a mechanism, an assembly of various sections.*
> *And it is not because the mechanism is working wrongly,*
> *That I am ill.*
> *I am ill because of wounds to the soul, to the deep emotional self*
> *And the wounds to the soul take a long, long time,*
> *Only time can help*
> *And patience, and a certain difficult repentance."*
>
> James Hollis

Shame, roots and illness

Q How did you embark on this journey of identifying wounding?

There were so many questions to be asked and to explore. To name a few:

- » What were the wounds?
- » Who wounded me?
- » When, where and how did the wounding take place?
- » How did it play out over the years?
- » What was the purpose of the wounding for this soul in this lifetime?

What I had thought was important, now seemed to be of little value and significance. It brought to mind a term in the Dictionary of Obscure Sorrows[20] – *avenoir*: the desire that memory could flow backward. According to the compositor, John Koenig, we take it for granted that life moves forward. But we move as a rower moves, facing backwards. We can see where we've been, but not where we're going.

I had to name the wounds and then work through them, and there were many. All the issues that I faced in later life were representative of issues around shame, abandonment and betrayal. When we feel shame about our roots, ourselves or our choices, speaking these truths amplifies the hidden universe. Until we can discharge our original shameful stories, we are held hostage by them, as they rob us of who we were meant to be. We sit in dark silence, possessed by our demons. Our inner turmoil is an expression of the lack of integration of the mind and the heart;

20 http://www.dictionaryofobscuresorrows.com

the lack of integration of the shadow of our lives against the larger canvas of our lives.

Addressing my wounding most certainly minimised the obstacles in my path to healing.

Whether the stressors are internal or external, they are life-sapping nonetheless. When unable to verbalise these stressors because of the shame associated with them, they became like a volcanic force that cannot abate, whose heat robbed me of the very water required to sustain the life force. I became a construct, an edited version of who I was meant to be, because I experienced the external world as threatening and the internal world as fragmented. And I could ill afford to open a septic wound without the skills to attend to it.

The incapacity of my illness drew me like a magnet to face and explore all aspects of the life I had lived, where people made me feel less than; unworthy of; not good enough to; the list goes on. The wounding came from a sense of not belonging, rooted in childhood, born of the stigma and shame I felt as the child of an intermarriage between a Jew and a gentile.

I began to explore illness as metaphor for blocked feelings trapped inside my body, creating tensions that had no avenues for release. My personal belief of not being good enough constricted the interaction between my inner and outer worlds. In a sense, we react to our environment and it reacts to us in an endless loop. My response to my shame increasingly drove me into isolation and solitude.

Q What story did the metaphor of your illness need to give a voice to?

The metaphor of my constricted voice lay hidden in my pelvic floor area. In Chinese medicine, pelvic floor muscles are associated with the muscles of longevity, and considered to act as the canary in the mine-shaft, alerting us to other medical issues in the body that may require healing. Western society is characterised by a way of life reflective of living in our minds, resulting in a loss of grounding connection with our bodies.

Grounding is essential because it is what roots and links us to wisdom, enabling us to stand erect and firm. It is in the pelvic basin, which is often disowned because of its association with our sense of shame, brought on by the wounding of which we do not speak. These secrets have their own destructive force, sapping us of psychic energy, leaving us depleted and feeling diminished, as we desperately try to hide them, as they continue to eat away bite by bite at our psyches and bodies.

Taking the concept of grounding further, the ancient Indian interpretation of energy systems is based on 'chakras', a Sanskrit word meaning wheel of life. Although many chakras spin within the human energy system, there are seven major chakras running from the base of the spine to the top of the head, each dealing with specific parts of the body and aspects of life and living.

The grounding chakra at the base of the spine is known as the 'mula bhanda'. Mula means root, foundation or origin. Bhanda means bondage or joining together. Mula bhanda is also referred to as 'the root lock' which prevents energy from leaking out of the body. This root chakra is believed to move energy up the centre of the body.

When we shine an Eastern light on Western attitudes, beliefs and thinking, it becomes clear that our culture and conditioning have moved our awareness away from being a whole person. For the most part, we grow up in homes where sex, bodily functions and many of our negative emotional responses are never discussed. We know instinctively that whatever we repress becomes a monster lurking in the darkness of our inner self. We know that it will express itself somehow.

The root chakra represents our stability, security and basic needs. The traumas and issues that create imbalances in this chakra then affect the tissues closest to that chakra – the pelvic floor.[21]

If illness was a metaphor of wounding of my psyche and soul, what part did culture play in this wounding? In addition, I wondered what the wounds were that I could refer to. My questions allowed me to have the courage to explore and own my story.

Initially I decided to explore the theme of shame in my life and illustrate its impact on my lived experience through sharing personal vignettes where wounding took place, and how it had unfolded.

Shame and intermarriage

Shame takes place in families or communities within the wider context of a culture. It stands to reason that shaming then is culture-specific. When we are in experience of having done something shameful, we conclude one of two things. The first is that "I messed up", the second is that "I am a mess." The former is an expression of guilt, the latter of shame.

Shame is the internalising of judgements held against us by others, leaving us feeling less worthy, not good enough, and so on. Shame is humiliating. When an individual chooses to marry a partner not of the same faith, their actions are a betrayal of the cultural norms and indirectly the culture itself. In turn, the culture shuns them, their actions, their choices and their chosen.

---

21 For more information on the connection between the root chakra and pelvic floor dysfunction, go to www.LisaFitzpatrick.com.au

Marrying someone of another culture may not be a value upheld by all cultures. In my grandparent's generation, it was not uncommon for the parents to rend their garments and sit shiva[22] symbolic of the death of the child who had chosen to defy cultural norms. You can well imagine what impact this must have had on both the child and the parents.

These are wounds that are indeed difficult to heal. But if you love someone and marry them despite cultural approval, it is a short-sighted step with long-lasting implications that are not considered at the time. Hence, we can only make sense of our choices in hindsight. The culture may choose to admonish this action by prohibiting the individual from participating in culturally sanctioned rites of passage or rituals.

Dr Mario Martinez, a clinical neuropsychologist and founder of the Bio Cognitive Science Institute, is a worldwide expert on how cultural beliefs impact health and longevity. He is of the opinion that our culture, beliefs, and immune systems all operate in a seamless unity, creating our experience of health. He asserts that many experiences within our culture serve to determine gene expression of wellness, or under-immunity (infections, cancer), over-immunity (allergies), and auto-immunity (rheumatoid arthritis, lupus). He cautions people never to blame themselves for their illness.

Martinez identifies three central archetypal wounds evident in all cultures: the wounds of abandonment, shame and betrayal.

---

22 An act of ritual mourning

Q Does Dr Martinez explain the links between the three types of wounding and specific illnesses?

The archetypal wound of abandonment has an adrenalin-based fight or flight response in the body, leaving the individual experiencing an immediate cold and fearful feeling. The primary disease linked to the wound of abandonment is cancer.

When an individual experiences betrayal, the fight or flight response is engendered in the body, releasing adrenalin and cortisol. However, the immediate response experienced by the individual is heat and anger. The disease correlated with the wounding of betrayal is heart disease.

Martinez believes that love can heal and transform all relationships.

When individuals experience feelings of ridicule, blame, judgment and criticism, being attacked and humiliated, they will experience the wounding of shame. Because the body feels like it is being attacked, the likely disease link to this kind of wounding would be a pro-inflammatory response to being cut or having an infection, and the disease link then is that of auto-immune diseases.

Q So let's focus on the wounding of your personal experience through shame.

The information given here is a backdrop to one personal example of shame that I will be discussing as part of what I grappled with during my illness. And I have no doubt there are many varied versions of how this choice unfolds. So, to the reader, kindly note that the case study represents the unfolding of this issue in the life of one family of origin and one family member. It does not necessarily reflect that this will be the road that will be walked by all people who marry out of their faith.

Martinez notes that fear of being shamed by our family and/or our culture is a strong determinant in who we choose to marry. Modern western society is characterised by high rates of assimilation and intermarriage, with Jewish divorce rates steadily reflecting those of the dominant culture. As children, we are socialised that this marrying within our faith is a strong cultural value and therefore not something that should be entertained lightly. The wound of shame becomes systemic in its impact, affecting both the parents and their children and the people they choose to partner through marriage.

As I contemplated all this and examined the role each played in my psyche, I came to the realization that to a greater or lesser extent, each of these wounds was part of me. And more importantly, these wounds needed personal healing.

> *Owning our story can be hard but not nearly as difficult as spending our lives running from it. Embracing our vulnerabilities is risky, but not nearly as dangerous as giving up on love and belonging and joy—the experiences that make us the most vulnerable. Only when we are brave enough to explore the darkness will we discover the infinite power of our light.*
>
> Brené Brown

This quote ignited my psychological journey, exploring one of my greatest woundings, that of shame. It was the shame associated with my identity, of my family of origin and my rejection by the community I identified with, the community I chose to belong to. I will draw on vignettes from my life to illustrate the theme of the convert and the shame associated with not belonging.

One day, sitting at my elder brother's bed, waiting for his approaching death, he looked up at me and said, "You know, I never really felt Jewish."

I stared at him, my mind reeling with my own understanding of his words. I thought he felt alienated from Jewish practice, had no understanding of its laws and customs, and was contemptuous in his perception of the shrinking minds of the ghetto. The lens through which he viewed the world was hazy, covered over with prejudice, indifference, contempt and projections of his own inadequacies. He had never contemplated a spiritual existence, let alone expressed any need for a spiritual path or journey. He was the proverbial secularist, and lived a life devoid of spiritual underpinnings. Although I did not respond to or query his comment, it struck a raw nerve in me. I wondered whether I could share the sentiment.

It is a difficult place to be when, as a Jew or a converted Jew, you feel alienated from the mainstream. It is a strange form of alienation when the people you pray with are not the people you can talk to. And the people you can talk to are not the people you can pray with. Many Jews experience this no man's land. Learning the laws of Shabbat[23] and kashrut[24] allows for an ease of expression in orthopraxy. It does not necessarily imply that they will enter the realms of spiritual connectedness to the G-d of Israel and, in turn, in shades of grey, shift their identity to the people whom G-d too had chosen.

23 The Jewish holy day of rest

24 The body of Jewish religious laws governing food and ritual objects

> *Before we can fully discover ourselves in community, we must discover who we are as individuals and to do that, we must know what lies at the depth of our soul.*
>
> Catherine Hall-Myerowitz

Religion and spirituality can often be experienced as a polarity. As we genuflect and mutter our prayers, do we ever feel a profound connection to the Divine, let alone to our fellow Jews? So to refer to the above quote, what is required is to discover first who we are as individuals and what lies at the depth of our souls before we can connect to community and to G-d. If we are disconnected from ourselves, how are we to connect to our fellow man, let alone the Divine?

The quality of the spiritual journey will ultimately be reflected in a deep and abiding sense of the Divine in our lives. Our lack of connection to organised religion may often be the result of deep wounding we have suffered as children and adults. And in our choice to belong and to convert, we bring these wounds with us. In the joining of our psyches with the psyches of our chosen group, we are often wounded once again.

> *Conversion is not the smooth, easy-going process some men seem to think… It is wounding work, this breaking of the hearts, but without wounding there's no saving… Where there is grafting there will always be cutting, the graft must be let in with a wound; to stick it onto the outside or to tie it on with a string would be of no use. Heart must be set to heart and back to back or there will be no sap from root to branch. And this, I say, must be done by a wound, by a cut.*
>
> John Bunyan

Conversion touches on the archetypal wounds of the psyche: shame, abandonment and betrayal. In our stories we wound and are wounded in all three spheres as we abandon, reject and are shameful of our roots as we dance the dance of silence around our abandoned and new identities. Then we enter the fold and are often in receipt of the same wounds, as if the test is to heal the very wounding we inflicted on others. This is a long and painful journey and requires awareness at a deep soul level of the journey undertaken and the cost thereof to the psyche and the soul.

As I mulled over my brother's comment, I wondered with a renewed sense of grief whether I had ever resolved the issues of identity. Born to a Jewish father and a gentile mother, the stage was set for polarity from the outset. But this polarity was to be no ordinary polarity; it was to be rooted in the spoils of war. Unable to resolve their issues around identity and joint identity, my parents chose the path of least resistance, the road of the unexamined life. It was going to be simple. The spoils of war would be divided equally and each would find comfort in their choices and their spoils. It was a simple move, predetermined, calculated and devoid of any consideration of the impact this choice would have on the spoils of their warring lives together. It was agreed, as if in the presence of Solomon, that if they had a daughter, she would be Christian and if they had sons, they would be Jewish. A win-win situation. And so began the journey.

My father was the eldest of nine children. His parents had left Bauska, due south of Riga, at the end of the nineteenth century. His father, Sheftel, and his brother, David had boarded a liner and landed sometime later in Cape Town to start a new life away from family and friends. It must have been a daunting undertaking indeed. My grandfather had a general dealership in Kirkwood, in the Eastern Cape and upon his death his obituary read:

Kirkwood News and Notes: Death of an old resident
Sunday 15.2.1936

The pioneer general dealer of the early days of the Sundays River Valley passed away on Saturday morning in the person of Mr Sheftel Liebowitz, at the age of 60 years. Arriving 40 years ago from Latvia, he established a general dealer and produce store and by his integrity and fair dealing won the esteem of everybody. When the Boer Commando under General Smuts raided the Valley, they commandeered stock giving him "good for" which were never redeemed. He was a founding member of the Kirkwood Village Management Board and a trustee of the Kirkwood Synagogue. The cortege left Kirkwood this morning for Port Elizabeth, where the burial rites were performed by Reverends Levy, Horwitz and Sandler.

My paternal grandmother, Gusta (nee Leventhal) birthed nine children, my father being the eldest and best beloved. She died tragically in a hit-and-run in 1956 when I was four years old, and is buried with my grandfather in Port Elizabeth.

The marriage of my father to my mother was fraught with shame, as intermarriage was considered taboo. For fear that my grandmother would sit shiva for him, my father did not tell his mother that he had married out of the faith, and that he had a son, whom my grandmother was not to meet until he was fourteen months old. Although a shock to my grandmother, she was not about to lose her best beloved. A year later, a second son was born. My father owned a hotel in Port Alfred. Their first-born child suffered from asthma and it was not long before his condition became life-threatening. My father sold the hotel, retired, and moved to Cradock in the Karoo, where the air was dry, the soil arid, the sun ablaze and the environment conducive to his son's health.

Alienation had crept into the marriage, and in this mix I was conceived. True to form, my mother snuck me away one Sunday morning to have me christened at a church in a nearby town. But the secret would soon reach my father's ears, and in a fit of rage he issued a new decree without consulting my mother. My father was the captain of his ship in a world where men ruled and women served. Yes, they served in many ways, some willingly and some unwilling. My mother fell into the latter category. My parents entered a time of silence, a cold war, which lasted until my father's death in 1980.

In 1958, the family moved from Cradock in the Eastern Cape to Bethlehem in the Orange Free State, a predominantly Afrikaans town. Growing up in a home where parents do not talk to each other, and in a hotel, which is not conducive to family life, was an arid environment indeed. It was about survival on every level. Mother took to running the kitchen and oversaw the running of the hotel. My father managed the administrative side of the hotel and took to socialising with the padres like a duck to water. My elder brother completed his schooling and left to study law at Wits, while my younger brother took over the family business after my father had a stroke. I was eleven years old.

This meant a sickly father who could no longer drive and an ever-angry mother left to take on more responsibilities. My father, my best friend and protector, disappeared before my eyes. My soul was literally convulsing with grief. Who would look after me now, I wondered.

Both my brothers had converted before me because I was the youngest in the family. But the spoils of war were still not his, so my father's attention turned to me, one of the two shiksas[25] left in the house. When you are the child of an intermarriage, derogatory comments about Jews and Christians strike a deep chord in you – because your identity is dual, as it your loyalty.

The younger of my brothers initiated a new round of arguments around my identity. "You are not Jewish and you need to convert," he lectured.

I was fifteen at the time and distraught at having to make this decision. It was not a decision about faith for me. It was a decision far deeper than that because it cut to the core of my identity and loyalty. Although I felt Jewish to my core, went to shul[26] on Shabbat, cheder[27] in the afternoons, enlisted for numerous habonim[28] camps and was sent to Israel on holidays at a young age to expose me to my roots, I was not ready for the spoils of war to be settled once and for all.

At school I was "die Joodjie[29]". With a name like Liebowitz, it was rather difficult to hide. The non-Jewish children had no problems with us. Once one slipped a Bible into my hand while walking down the corridor at school, only to disappear in to the crowds – she wanted to save my soul.

And so I reluctantly went to see Rabbi Altshuler and explained with tears running down my face that I did not want a certificate to prove that I was Jewish. That is what my father wanted. I explained the story of the spoils of war and urged him to relay this to my

---

25 A derogatory term for a non-Jewish woman

26 Synagogue

27 A school for Jewish children where they learn Hebrew and the fundamentals of the Jewish religion

28 A progressive Labour Zionist youth movement that emphasizes cultural Judaism, socialism and social justice

29 Afrikaans: The little Jew; a term meant to set you apart from others

father. When I was ready I would convert and become a practising Jew, as I saw no point in doing it for a piece of paper or to appease my father.

Not good enough: rejection of the shiksa

And so, the wounding around the shame of being a child of an intermarriage took on a life all of its own. I was not allowed to go to parties and date non-Jewish boys and in Bethlehem the Jewish boys were few and far between.

And so, it happened that I met a young Jewish man undergoing his military training at the Military Base in Bethlehem. When circumstances suit the agenda of the parents, the game plan changes very quickly. He came to us every Friday night for supper with a troop of other Jewish boys undergoing their military training. We took an instant liking to one another and formed a relationship of trust and repartee over the remaining year. When he left at the end of his training I was preparing for my matric examinations.

My father had booked an overseas trip for me to Europe, and it was agreed that I would fly up to Johannesburg and stay with my friend and his parents for a few days before flying out to Lisbon. His parents were delighted to see me and made me most welcome.

He was the eldest of three boys. One afternoon his brother had to be picked up from the cricket field at Wanderers, and his mother asked me to join her for the drive. While waiting in the car, she initiated a discussion.

"Does your elder brother have a girlfriend and has your father met her?" It took me a few seconds to realize where I thought this conversation was heading. My brother had a non-Jewish girlfriend at the time. I felt rising discomfort within me and responded to it.

"My brother does have a non-Jewish girlfriend and yes, my father has met her. I think what you are asking me is whether my mother is Jewish or not."

She had not expected such a direct response.

"Well, is she?" she asked.

"No, my mother is Christian and never converted to Judaism. But my brothers have converted," I replied.

She burst into tears realising that she was in the car talking to her eldest son's girlfriend, the shiksa. What followed haunted me for years.

"I am so ashamed of you and I do not want my husband to find out about this," she said, her voice rising as she spoke.

I was young and innocent. Shame welled up in me and I knew in that instant that I was not good enough. We drove home in silence and the following day I left for Lisbon. I had shared nothing of the conversation with my friend. I telephoned him many times from overseas, but he never took my calls.

On my return, my brother drove me past his house and dropped me off to visit him and pick up my things. I knocked on the door. It opened and there he stood. He showed me to the lounge, me following with gifts for him and the family. I was immediately overcome by the enormity of silence and heaviness in the house.

"Where is the family?" I asked.

"They're in their bedrooms," he explained.

"Sit down, I have something to say to you," he said uncomfortably. "I have two thousand years of Jewish blood running through my veins. You cannot be in this house because you are not Jewish."

He showed me to the door and we walked around the suburb for the remaining two hours. I shared my trip with him, but we spoke little of what had just transpired. When my brother arrived, I was waiting with my case in hand and climbed into the car. Then the sobbing began. My brother was enraged. And so began the journey of the wound called shame.

I returned to my rooms to lick my wounds and decided that my avoidance of conversion had reached critical mass. I was going to have to make the choice I had always wanted to make and find some way to deal with the hurt and the grief that this was going to cause my mother. I dialled her number and waited for her to answer.

"Ma, I have decided to convert and I need you to sign the forms because I am under age," I explained.

"I won't sign them," she responded.

The telephone went dead. I thought about this for a few days and telephoned again.

"Ma, I am going to convert and if you do not sign the forms you will no longer be my mother. This is your and dad's war, not mine. I have had enough. And I am tired of being in the middle like I've been for the past eighteen years. I need to find my own path." There was a long pause.

"Okay, I will sign them, my child," she answered.

The shiksa's daughter had to decide about her identity. I was never going to subject myself to such shaming ever again. But this was not to be the case. I approached the Beth Din and requested to convert to Judaism.

"Are you involved with someone?" one asked.

"No," I responded. "What I want is to convert and live with a religious Jewish family and would like you to arrange this for me."

It was near my third-year examinations and I lived on my own in a small room in a hotel in Hillbrow and I would walk to Wits each day. As exams neared, I had taken to studying at the central library in town. On one such day at lunch time I took a break. Upon my return, I chose to change seats and seated myself near a pile of books that someone had used and left behind.

Suddenly someone stood next to me. He was wearing a yarmulke[30] and asked if he could sit down. I beckoned to him because there was plenty of space.

Shame and betrayal: inclusion factors, marriage and commitment

As things transpired, some two years later the young man I had met at the library proposed to me. I was to learn from bitter experience that I was too naïve to discern what was beneath the mask of religiosity. I had entered a world I lacked the coping skills to handle. I was swirling in confusion and had no one to talk to. How does one talk about the state of affairs in a new marriage without the deepest sense of shame?

In desperation eight years later, I went to see a psychologist who was the Professor of Psychology at Jerusalem University. This was the beginning of my disillusionment with Judaism, as I found it difficult to divorce the two. Had I just married the wrong man or had I chosen the wrong path? Was this my punishment for the punishment meted out to my mother through my choice to convert? In my last session with the psychologist I asked him what advice he would give me if I was his daughter.

"If you were my daughter Leah, I would tell you to pack your bags and run," he said.

It took a total of seventeen years to pack my bags and flee the life I had chosen and chosen badly.

30 Skull cap

Shame: conversion, belonging and indifference

> *The basic dynamics of conversion are summed up for me in the words*
> ***LEAVE – ARRIVE,***
> ***END – BEGIN,***
> ***SHED – EMERGE.***
> *These are the tensions of conversion and spiritual awakening.*
>
> Sue Monk Kidd

The process of conversion, culminating in final acceptance, can be fraught with many emotions, but none can prepare you for the rejection by Jews once you have converted.

Confronting the firmly entrenched prejudice that Jews are born and not made is something I experienced over the years. When my mother died in 1991, the father of my children did not attend her funeral. When I returned home and took it upon myself to sit shiva, her death was not acknowledged and no comfort arrived. So there was religion and religious laws, but a glaring lack of compassion.

You see, you don't have to mourn the loss of a shiksa, because mourning rituals do not apply to her. And so I was surprised when my colleagues popped by and the first thing one of them blurted out, to my utter amazement, was, "You foxed us, didn't you? We thought that you were Jewish!"

Nineteen years had passed since my conversion. Who were these people, I wondered. In an instant, I had once again become the ger[31], a thinly played script. I was to learn in years to come that when you leave the tribe, you pay a price. But the price you pay when you stay with the tribe is even greater.

---

31 A convert

Nietzsche revisited – making sense of duality

One morning I woke up to the sounds of my mother singing. I had never heard my mother sing before. It was 1985 in Jerusalem and my mother had come to visit. She was singing a song of praise about the Lord. Gingerly, I tiptoed towards the doorway. There I could see her sitting in bed and heard the following conversation.

"Nachon[32] Safta[33], when you sing to the Lord, you are singing to Hashem?" Yael my first-born daughter asked. "Oh no," said my mother. "I am singing to the Lord, the Son of Hashem."

In her simplicity Elisheva, my younger daughter, aged 4 at the time, looked on in bewilderment and blurted out, "You mean the daddy died?"

Lineage from the mouths of babes

I was walking my daughters home from school one day when we got to talking about religion.

"Nachon Ima[34]," Yael said, "You were not born Jewish?"

"Yes," I said. "Does that confuse you?"

"Yes, it does."

"What do you think I am?" I asked.

"I think, Ima, you are both."

32 It is true

33 Grandmother

34 Mother

Shame and wounding

Q So what is your understanding of wounding?

Dr Mario Martinez points out that all cultures (East and West) have their own unique ways of punishing those whose ideas and behaviours run contrary to established beliefs and norms. Punishment for transgression of these cultural norms is transmitted from parents to children and becomes particularly evident when we fall in love and choose to marry. The community and family's response to what they may view as betrayal will evoke punishment of the couple with resultant psychological damage which surfaces as wounds, in my instance, the archetypal wound of shame. He calls these wounds archetypal because they are consistent across cultures.

Martinez uses the term 'cultural editors' to describe persons important in your culture or context who mirror the feedback that you are not who you believe yourself to be. Their devaluation of your character and worth becomes incorporated into your sense of self-worthiness. So when as a child, the feedback is that you are not worthy of love and belonging, the child's self-image is formed in relation to feedback from their family, community and tribe.

In later life, the nervous system and endocrine system respond to any positive feedback by experiencing it as a compromised sense of self-worthiness, precisely because it does not resonate with the subjective sense of self rooted in their history. So if someone important in your life tells you that you are worthy, but your inner belief is that you are unworthy, you will be unable to acknowledge the compliment because your inner world does not resonate with the message based on early wounding of being devalued or never receiving positive affirmation.

Martinez notes that we have a very selective perception based on our neuromaps (neural pathways) of who we are. Is it therefore possible that we unconsciously seek out contexts that affirm our inner worth based on our history. In other words, if we have experienced shame in our growing years, we will be more drawn to contexts that are shaming than to contexts that affirm our sense of self. Do we unconsciously replay the wounding over and over again?

People whose histories are clouded with trauma or negative experiences are unable to integrate positive experiences with ease. Positive experiences begin to feel like turbulence and they default to negative contexts or experiences. Only once the person is able to fully internalise their own sense of worthiness are they able to break the negative patterns rooted in toxic histories or toxic environments.

Cultures inform you about what you can and cannot accept. So a culture that does not allow outsiders to join them would have a specific view on outsiders and would make it more difficult for outsiders to join their ranks, if at all. So what happens when you join a culture that rejects the outsider and your wounding is rooted in shame and belonging to this particular culture? How does one help people like that? Martinez believes that it is vital to identify the cultural wounding, for example, "You were abandoned therefore you're not worthy."

We are co-authors of our lives, the wounds and the instance of shame, and we have to be able to develop an honour consciousness. This is a gradual process, but in time the feeling of lack of self-worthiness begins to change, and is replaced by a sense of worthiness. The shifting of consciousness requires retrieving memories and expressing some of those negativities, so that the languaging of shame can be replaced by the languaging of honour.

Q Is it possible to heal from this?

You learn to create contexts in which you do not hurt yourself or anybody else. It requires that you set boundaries for how you are prepared to be treated. Martinez refers to this as benign limits.

A person who is able to focus on the healing field of their particular wounding can shift their self-worthiness and empowerment. And like all shifts, it takes time. When you repeat something, it creates more neural pathways. If your neuromap is one of negativity, it will take time, commitment and inner work to bring about the tendency towards health, rather than illness. The body is constantly defaulting to health. Genetics is only 5–10 percent.

Culture can most definitely create biology. A good example of this is seen in how two cultures view menopause. Peruvian culture calls the hot flashes *borchorno,* which is another word for shame. When Peruvian women are tested for interleukins and other inflammatory products, the levels are high. In Japan, menopause is viewed as a woman's 'second spring', an opportunity for wisdom. Their inflammatory products are normal.

> *To live without love, compassion, or any other spiritual value creates a state of such severe imbalance that every cell yearns to correct it. Ultimately, that is what lies behind the onset of disease; the body is sending a message that something lacking in the present – an imbalance existing somewhere – has given rise to highly visible, unarguable, physical symptoms.*
>
> Deepak Chopra

Throughout history cultures have attempted to oust those whom they view as dark and have incorporated ways in their ceremonies and rites to do just that. These ceremonies serve the useful purpose of ridding the community of perceived or actual evil within its midst, in a cleansing ritual. In Leviticus, similar reference is made to the Yom Kippur service.

The Jewish Day of Atonement is ushered in by the sacrifice of two goats. This holy day and its associated rituals are profound in the religious life of the tribe. The sacrifice performed by the high priest on behalf of the community allows for the pardoning of their sins and the development of a new consciousness going forward. The people have come out of their own wilderness to seek atonement and thereby return once again to the tribe and to their G-d unblemished, ready to recommit to a new cycle, a new way of being in the world.

The Hebrew word for purification is *kippurim*, and involves ways to purge communities of that which is repressed or expelled. In the original Hebrew text, the priest is the agent of the collective, the one who approaches G-d on behalf of the community to atone for their sins. He is the mediator between the earthly and the mystical realms.

In the first part of the ritual the priest approaches the Holy of Holies and atones for his family and himself. In the second part, the dedication of the goats commences. Two goats are set aside, representing the Divine realm and the human realm. One goat is used as a sin offering, in atonement for the sins of the children of Israel. The goat is then killed and its blood is used to cleanse the sanctuary, including its contents such as the altar. Its blood serves to atone for the sins of Israel and the goat's remains are treated as defiled and burned outside the camp.

The second goat, the scapegoat, is herded off into the wilderness once the high priest has atoned for the transgressions, faults and sins of the community. Through this action, the goat wanders into the wilderness, carrying the collective guilt of the community, symbolically restoring the community's sense of integrity.

Q What is your understanding of the link between tribal wounding and illness?

Tribal wounding involves the rejection and expulsion of a tribal member. I am of the opinion that issues around identity (family, community, neighbourhood, spiritual community, national identity) play a role in the psyche of those in experience of shame, increasing the likelihood that illness as metaphor will present itself in areas of the body correlated energetically with issues of shame. If tribal or family wounding affected your sense of belonging resulting in feelings of estrangement, rejection and shaming, then this is relevant in the illness of narrative. I am not surprised, given the strength of patriarchy that women suffer from pelvic floor prolapse.

Tribes are important to human beings because they ensure identity, define beliefs and mores, provide protection in times of vulnerability and ensure safety and survival for its members. But all of this is conditional based on the degree to which the individual subscribes to the ethos of the tribe. A valued member of the tribe abides by the tribes rules. If you betray the tribe, the emotional and physical severance that follows will single you out for lack of loyalty precisely because you are viewed as a threat. Should you, in your naiveté, return to the tribe, they will make your life unbearable because they will interpret this as weakness? Because the tribe has authority, its members know full well that in order to *belong,* they need to speak with one tribal voice, lest they too become the outsiders, relegated to wandering the deserts.

We ascribe meaning through our connections, whether personal or tribal. We define who we are in relation to the tribe and through action adhere to its mores, rituals and rules. Our tribal values, beliefs and rules determine and impact on our choices, prejudices, values and what we consider sacred or profane. All of these serve to hold the tribe together in a living organismic state of cohesion, conformity and continuity. The path we are to walk, the way we are to walk and the direction and destination towards which we walk … all prescribed by the tribe. Strict adherence ensures our safety. Lack of adherence is akin to psychic annihilation.

There are families by blood (those we were born into) and there are families of choice (those like-minded folk with whom we share our faith, dreams, desires and journey). Many people experience dissonance with the tribe's ethos. They walk to a different drum beat, they talk a different language, they sing a different song and their values are not those of the tribe. Their vision is altered precisely because they walk the periphery of the tribe, allowing them to view the world and its interactions from a different vantage point. This is how the tribe scapegoats those who choose to walk alone, risking their lives and often on the receiving end of extreme acts of visible and sometimes invisible violence.

Most times the tribe uses shame, a more subtle form of violence, but more deadly in its wounding. In fact, shaming a person is the most powerful tool a tribe has at its disposal. It is a collective shaming, brutal in its onslaught, decisive in its wounding. Shame is their way of ostracising you from the collective. And they will use this over and over compulsively; they are unable to look at themselves or own their shadow aspects so they take on a godlike stance of judgement towards others, meting out their legalistic lashings one by one. How pitiful they are. They can destroy your identity, your psyche, and rob you of your name through their acts of cruelty. If you could be a fly on the wall in many therapists' consulting rooms you would be privy to relentless and ongoing tales of scapegoating and the damage it does. All these tales are kept hidden by an ethical code of conduct. The tribal machinations are silenced once again in the service of psychic healing. Tribal shame ruins lives, families, individuals. Some even take their own lives when the shaming becomes too much.

This brings to mind the quote by Alexander Solzhenitsyn in his book *The Gulag Archipelago*, where he notes:

> *If only it were all so simple! If only there were evil people somewhere, insidiously committing evil deeds, and it were necessary only to separate them from the rest of us and destroy them. But the line dividing good and evil cuts through the heart of every human being. And who is willing to destroy a piece of his own heart?*

When we stand by and diminish the value of one life, lash by lash, are we any better than a predator that eats away at its prey while it is still alive? It is the victory of our animal soul over our godly soul when man does such things. In modern times the Holocaust is an example of man's inhumanity to man, calculated without compassion, enacted with dedicated precision, sanctioned by the need for tribal purity.

Who are we? What are we capable of?

Martinez points out that even though they delegate you to the wilderness to die, if you fail in the wilderness they will always welcome you back. They have far more difficulty welcoming you back if you become successful. Unconsciously, many of those in the wilderness fail precisely because they cannot survive without their connection to a tribe.

What a tribute to human potential to restore our sense of belonging by returning to the tribe. That tribe may be a constellation of friends, neighbours, colleagues, team members, political parties, church affiliations and so on. No matter the composition of the tribe, even if made up of outsiders, the outcast and forsaken, they all have the propensity to emulate the wounding and excommunicate you from the tribe.

The same way illness may be seen as a transformative experience, is it at all possible that shaming may have a similar result? Could scapegoating be a gift in some perverse way?

Martinez spends a lot of time working with people who have left their tribes of origin for reasons ranging from deviation from the norm to being too successful. The term used in common parlance for this is the *Tall Poppy Syndrome*, a pejorative term denoting a social phenomenon in which people of genuine merit are cut down, criticised and devalued because their gifts and successes make them stand out in the crowd. They do not fit the norm nor do they wish to.

Shame, rejection, exile and healing

Q **So how is shame healed over time?**

Shame requires an energy field of honour. Only when you are able to arrive at that still point of honour, is the healing complete.

- What was the relationship between my archetypal shame and the tribe that I chose to belong to?
- In which way does childhood wounding play itself out in later life?
- What was the price paid to join the tribe?
- What was the price to leave the tribe?
- What happens to converts who are wounded by the tribe they joined?

The mark of children of intermarriage is alienation, a sense of living in a no-man's land, a land of dual identity, a land of lack. The very issue of identity confusion requires a solution of conscious choice to identify and align oneself with a particular group or community. This can be a community of like-minded individuals or a community of faith.

My childhood experience of dual identity had a marked impact on my psyche as well as my identification with belonging to a specific community in later life. The issue of faith was never really resolved, but underpinning this was a lack of belonging, of feeling like the eternal outsider.

My childhood familiarity with the outsider role seemed to roll over into my adult life. In retrospect, my understanding of this may be rather simplistic, but I shall attempt to explain it in a way that makes sense to me.

The core issue of the outsider – the black sheep of the family, the scapegoated or the child who is the index patient coming for therapy, symbolising or carrying the systemic concerns within the family – is feeling peripheral to the collective, whether this is the family or the community. This wounding that we carry with us, often unconsciously, is what drives most of our behaviour in later life, often replaying these wounds in other contexts. So if we feel unwanted, unloved, blemished in some way, I am of the opinion that the wounding unconsciously propels us to contexts where we replay the old scripts of being the outsider, the victim, the blemished one, the maverick, the one who does not share the vision of the tribe.

These souls are drawn, if not driven, to sabotage this sense of belonging, to become the outsider because deep down we are more at home in discomfort than we are in comfort, whether emotional or psychological. Deep down, the wound is never totally healed.

I am of the opinion that Christianity in its most complex and simplistic view of unconditional acceptance and forgiveness of all men, is a worldview or faith that allows the blemished, the fallen, the broken and the outsiders to feel loved and worthy of belonging despite their past. It is inclusive in its faith and connection to its followers. You can be a criminal and still be worthy of forgiveness and redemption. By definition it is not exclusive.

The Hebrew scapegoat

> *Judgement is mine, saith the Lord.*
>
> Hebrews 10:30

This brings me back to the sacrificial goat and its symbolism. Individuals cast out by community are like the sacrificial goat that is sent out into the wilderness, as a token of the blemished part of the community, symbolic of the rejected and unacceptable attributes with which they do not wish to identify.

These individuals or groups are often accused of causing misfortune to and within the community. By banishing them from the life of community, the community is able to regain homeostasis; its belief that they are cleansed through the expulsion of that which is undesirable.

If we can identify a scapegoat, it relieves us of our transpersonal relationship to G-d. If we can rid ourselves of the scapegoat, we are able to heal the community.

Who are these scapegoats?

Scapegoats come in many shapes and forms. Those who are perceived to be a threat to community cohesion are easily identified as scapegoats. All they need to do is break the silence of tribal myths, expose the unspoken darkness within the community or cause chaos within existing community structures. The tribe or community has no other way to deal with the imbalance or exposure of underlying myths and transgressions than to relieve themselves of this darkness through scapegoating, thereby strengthening their sense of power and sense of self-righteousness.

The voices have been silenced. The invisible acts of violence against the scapegoat are forgotten and unacknowledged. The community narrative remains intact with no quisling threatening its 'truth' or undermining its deception.

What happens if the scapegoats wish to return? Is their banishment to the wilderness more compassionate than what the community would do to them if they remained?

This delegation to the wilderness is actually the saving grace of the person being scapegoated. In their cruelty they have done the scapegoated individual a great favour. The wilderness symbolises that place which is disconnected from the main, that landscape of inhospitable brutal aridness no man is expected to survive. It is a form of a death sentence to banish someone to such a place.

But herein lies the beauty of the act, almost as if G-d in his infinite compassion, blesses the scapegoat on his journey forward. In the perceived suffering of abandonment, admonishment and annihilation lies the gold needed for the healing. The wilderness experience in its starkness is more life affirming than is the tribe or the community doing the abandoning. The wilderness is where we confront the unknown, our aloneness, our loneliness, the otherness that makes us unique in G-d's plan for our life.

There is no better place to know G-d than when we are in the desert. Herein lies the gift. This drawing closer to the Divine would not have been possible in the collective. The perceived communal abandonment is ultimately replaced by the realisation that G-d is all they have and need. What a powerful alliance.

The wilderness becomes a safe haven because the rejection and admonishments have wounded the scapegoat. The rejection and victimisation result in fear of connection or closeness to others lest they suffer more shame, betrayal and rejection. In modern parlance, it is an experience akin to post traumatic stress disorder. The wilderness lends itself to lack of connection, culminating in a defensive stance, the individual ever waiting for a replay of the original wounding.

We need to get past this defensiveness to discover our true selves in the wilderness.

Where then do we find these individuals? Which communities do they belong to? Does anyone ever wish to acknowledge them?

Or are they forever banished to the wilderness searching for water, as they come upon oasis after oasis, forever having to confront the illusion of unconditional love, safety, belonging and resolved identity?

Is their healing possible?

> *Be around the light chasers;*
> *The magic makers, the world shifters, the game shakers.*
> *They challenge you, break you open,*
> *Uplift and expand you.*
> *They don't let you play small with your life.*
> *These heartbeats are your people.*
> *These people are your tribe.*
>
> Anonymous

These individuals are blessed because ultimately they are drawn to like-minded wounded healers, fellow sufferers who smooth balm on their weary souls, fellow travellers seeking to help heal those who bear the mark of Cain, those who suffer, those who walk this earth in psychic pain.

This raises the interesting question of how the healing takes place. Scapegoated individuals are readily willing to take on suffering. They have a remarkable ability to witness, endure and risk change. While the complex can be managed, it will never disappear.

Q What then do they tend to do with their inner suffering?

Usually this is expressed in the form of creativity or entering a healing discipline. Hence the term 'wounded healer'. The scapegoat's inclination to live on the outskirts of the community enables them to cope with intensities that other people don't have the wherewithal to withstand. Scapegoats often become the healers within the contexts in which they received their wounding. Because they have a renewed sense of wholeness, they are able to assist others in attaining their wholeness. So there is an ongoing dance between the healer and the wounded, an interchange through which both are healed.

Q How do we know when the wounding has been resolved?

Initially, the scapegoat can see only those unacceptable parts of themselves identified by the scapegoater. The scapegoater has seen in the scapegoat their own shadow, because, as the saying goes, "If you've got it, you spot it."

Scapegoats need to see the gold in their own darkness and bring it into the light of their everyday lives, slowly, bit by bit until the identity the scapegoater assigned them is no longer all they can see of themselves. They become less and less akin to that identity as they revisit and own their unique place in the world and their unique contribution, no matter what it is. As their self-concept slowly changes away from the scapegoating context, they become incisive in their understanding of the world and the players in the worldly and cosmic drama of their wounding. Now the scapegoater and the scapegoat speak a different language, belong to different tribes, and reside in different realities.

These are the very people who commit to a life-long search for personal growth and the growth of others. So in my instance, the withdrawal led to profound realisations during the period of illness and forced me into writing, a creative side of me not tapped into before with the same intensity. Illness serves as the catalyst for rectification and revisiting the underbelly, the dark, unconscious aspects of our selves and the tribe we chose to leave.

In my journal entry under the title *Blowing out someone else's candle does not make yours burn brighter*, I caution individuals to refrain from letting others define who you are, whether through scapegoating, minimising your success or projecting their own inadequacies:

> *I tried, failed often and achieved much, and when the losses and gains were audited, I realised that I had showed up and taken my rightful place.*
>
> *Surviving nonetheless, myself intact, my worth restored, my shame diminished, and my honour regained.*
>
> *No longer do I listen to their derogatory howling as they confront their own shortcomings, critics, demons and capacity for cruelty.*
>
> *For the lives they stole, names they blemished, murders committed if only in name. Their time will come, their deeds will be audited, reckoning will be held for the deeds done in malice, sans thought.*
>
> *Like ravaging animals gnawing at their live prey while it writhes, bleeds, fights for its life, gasps for air and dies.*
>
> *Don't wash your blood-stained hands or cover them with gloves.*
>
> *Reveal your blood-stained hands like Cain wore his mark, so that others may know what you are capable of and you never forget who you essentially are.*

Q What did the wounding force you confront in terms of your life's meaning?

To this day, I struggle with forgiveness in relationship to these acts. Clearly, the work is not yet done.

I grappled intensely with my life's purpose, sensing acutely that it had something to do with the awakening of the consciousness of others. But first I had to rise from my own slumber and waken to the call I had failed to heed so many times.

Writing, teaching and support were going to be the medium through which this illness would transmute me. Change was inevitable. Never was I to underestimate who I believed I was meant to be at this juncture. Slowly the realisation dawned on me that I needed a voice, but I was not sure where it would speak and to whom, let alone the medium. But the window period was narrow indeed. I felt vulnerable and believed in my protection. Only time would prove which way the dice would fall.

I had a sense that I had only achieved half of what needed to be achieved. And achievement could take on many forms. It may even be being able to tell someone that you love them on the day of their death. There were many achievements left for this fractured soul. I would have to wait patiently to embrace my health and the relentless pain. It was a slow process, but life would one day return to normal.

At 64, five surgeries later, I came to the realisation that, above all, I was worthy of love and belonging. This profound knowing and the internalisation of this truth allowed me to regain my sense of power.

Q How do you understand the concept of the wilderness that Jung refers to?

Jung contends that the wilderness represents a feeling of never belonging, a lack of internal safety and a lack of self-acceptance. In its most extreme form, individuals may wish for death to end this anguish. In this scapegoating and rejection lies the seed of one's healing, the gold lies in the dark so to speak.

What on earth does this mean? When we are in the wilderness, far away from the sounds of distraction of the modern world, we are brought to a still point where we are better able to discern the incessant inner chatter. This is the time for recognition of the level of discordance within our lives. It is time out of time, a place where the unconscious is able to meet the conscious and in doing so provide the grounding for the healing to begin.

As in the period of my illness, the time out of time experience from community is beyond valuable. It begs for the exploration of the unfinished work, the dark elements that needed acknowledgement, the wounds that needed healing, the fractured relationships that needed mending.

It begs for our ownership of our lived experience, both the dark and light, and it calls for a commitment to the rectification of those times when we have inadvertently betrayed ourselves, our fellow humans or our God. This is a profound journey. It calls for ruthless honesty, for humility, for compassion for others and ourselves, for the grieving of the past and the resurrection of the new. In a nutshell it calls for a transformation of who we were, who we are and a commitment to who we were meant to be.

Q What purpose does the wounding serve in our psychic development?

A 'wounded healer' is one who as a function of having transformed his wounding, develops a psychological capacity "to be at home in the darkness of suffering and there to find germs of light and recovery…[35]". Transformation calls for an altered perception of why the wounding happened in the first place, who sanctioned it, why you were chosen to be wounded, and what the wounding achieved.

The wounding is to be reframed as an invitation to interact with the wounded part of ourselves, embracing and owning it nonetheless, and redefining ourselves as whole despite the initial wounding. It calls for revisiting the enactment of the wounding over time, and requires resilience, honesty, ownership, transparency, patience, courage and forgiveness of ourselves and others.

Our wound is a continually unfolding dynamic process, a work in progress, pointing us towards the gold (healing, calling, getting back on track with our soul's purpose) that lies in the dark (wound itself). The mere exploration, ownership and embracing of ourselves as we are, is part of the healing. The initial chains that bound us and imposed restrictions, even if self-imposed, are released, and in so doing invite a new narrative to unfold.

It is an initiation experience, a shedding of the skin of the old self and a resurrection and rebirth of the new self. In the simplest yet most profound terms, it is a rebirth of psychic and quantum proportions.

---

35 Quote from Karl Kerényi, a peer of Carl Jung

Jung's rendition and commentary on the story of Jacob wrestling with the angel reflects in a nutshell the essence of this transformation.

When we encounter a force (the angel) greater than ourselves and our ego (the self), we are forever transformed. Jacob (the supplanter) wrestles with the angel, and at daybreak finds himself wounded on his hip by the angel's touch. This kind of initiatory wounding by a force greater than ourselves is transforming to such an extent that we experience a rebirth of sorts. The Jacob who lay down to rest is not the Jacob who awoke in the morning – so much so that his name was changed from Jacob to Israel (he who has wrestled with G-d), symbolic of a new identity.

The wounding is G-d's way of connecting with Jacob in this drama of life. It is a wounding that serves as a rectification, in my humble opinion, of a soul's journey in need of redirection.

Another way of looking at the struggle is to view it as a struggle between two sides of Jacob, the shadow and the integrated parts of his being. What Jacob needs to confront is that both of these sides are part of him. It calls for an acceptance of self not entertained until that moment.

Once he is able to transform through reintegrating all aspects of himself, he is able to release that shameful identity and face the meeting with his brother head on.

The more powerful the archetypal forces that wound us, the greater the challenge to intimately acquaint ourselves with the more empowered aspects of ourselves. The perceived obstructive wounding of ourselves by others leaves us feeling isolated. However, within this isolation, this feeling of disconnection from others, this relegation to the wilderness, lies the seed of the awakening of our potential and destiny. Separation from the whole seems to be one aspect of the transformative process. Separation brings loneliness, aloneness, searching, lack of connection. Maybe these are important experiences to encounter in the journey back to ourselves, precisely because the wounding is part of a Divine cosmic drama, a portal through which we enter a vista of potential purpose and shift in our identity.

Q How do you make sense of all of this in retrospect?

> *Many people are born into their religion. For them it is mostly a matter of legacy and convenience. Their belief is based on faith, not just in the teachings of the religion but also in the acceptance of that religion from their family and culture. For the person who converts, it is a matter of fierce conviction and defiance. Our belief is based on a combination of faith and logic because we need a powerful reason to abandon the traditions of our families and community to embrace beliefs foreign to both. Conversion is a risky business because it can result in losing family, friends and community support.*
>
> Kareen Abdul-Jabbar

In retrospect, I now have a better understanding of why the process of conversion, its wounding and associated shame, was such a painful experience for me. I have come to the point where I have greater acceptance of the impact it had on my lived experience. The shame and the blame I experienced around this has been replaced by the knowledge that it took courage, commitment and fortitude to undertake the journey; a journey that encompassed great wounding in a tribal context. This was a personal journey and does not necessarily reflect the journey of other converts.

What started for me as an issue of not being good enough, being disconnected from the mainstream, an outsider, became an enlightening and extraordinary journey.

From seeing the shame, abandonment and betrayal as personal wounding, I am now able to see the transpersonal nature of all that has unfolded. The struggle made me undertake an exploration of old wounding, which ultimately led me to invest in my creativity, which had hitherto remained dormant. This transformation gave me invaluable insights into what healing really is. It gave me the ability to sit with my pain and the pain of others and to entertain a future from a completely different perspective, if not from another realm of understanding.

In effect, the transformation was the refining of the wounded-healer aspects of my being. I am fascinated by how it was through the illness and withdrawal from the pulse of living that the search commenced, culminating in a destination vastly different from the intended destination.

I realise now that our wounding and our healing are unique to each one of us. Yet, at the same time, it is a process that invites so many players to participate unwittingly and unconsciously. When we are in experience of self, both as a personal and transpersonal experience towards wholeness, we awaken our consciousness. We become intimately aware of the outside world and how it impacts on our inner world. The two are intertwined.

The outer destructive forces in our lives have a way of activating and triggering processes within ourselves, giving rise to our subjective experiences of our wound. The wound therefore contains the medicine required for our healing. It is both our personal problem as well as a quantum phenomenon, uniquely tailored for each of us, to bring about a desired outcome. The wound is not separate from the psyche in experience of it. The wound also reflects that part of us that is not wounded. It takes wounding to recognise the aspects of ourselves that have not been wounded. The wound comes to represent the wholeness that existed prior to the wounding, and which, once the healing takes place, we become again. But we would never have arrived at this place without the specific wounding unique to ourselves.

Everything is interconnected. It is only the conceptual mind that distinguishes between us and them. As we become conscious of this fact and the opposites that exist in our lives, we are in experience of our wholeness – embracing all of who we are, without apology, yet in awe.

Q Is it possible that genital surgery could trigger unresolved issues in our personal history?

Many aspects of wounding and its associated shame experienced by women remain invisible. I think that pelvic floor surgery touches on an aspect of our lives that is deeply personal, deeply private, deeply sacred, often scarred. It can and does reveal wounds that have often been buried for so long that we have long forgotten them and are confused by the feelings that may surface.

Those memories, those traumas hidden from view, those promises not kept, betrayals not healed – all of these can be brought to the surface by surgery. Any trauma, whether surgical or a life trauma can trigger a state of deep vulnerability in patients, releasing deep emotions related to previous unresolved losses and wounding.

There is wounding from the past and there is wounding that takes place in the present and both have to be dealt with as a parallel process. The wounds may be psychological, physical, sociological or spiritual in origin, but they exist nonetheless and have a psychic force of their own.

But deep down I know that this is the beginning of a journey not a place of arrival. The question for me then is, after all that has gone before, how would my interactions in the world differ as a function of the healing? How will I walk, talk, connect and belong in a way that tangibly shows that the shifts have taken place? The surgery and the illness brought with it its own challenges and wounding which invited, if not forced me to deal with emotions, realisations and challenges I had not faced before.

Shame, gender, pelvic organ prolapse and surgery

Q You speak of the shame associated with pelvic floor dysfunction. Could you extrapolate on the kinds of unvoiced shame that you experienced?

> *All of us feel shamed by life. All of us consider ourselves failures of some kind, screw ups in something really important to us. Notice how shame consciously pulls us away from risk, ratifies our negative sense of worth through self-sabotage or compels us into frenetic efforts of overcompensation or yearning for the validation from others that never comes; how much each of us needs to remember one definition of grace as accepting the fact that we are accepted despite the fact that we are unacceptable.*
>
> James Hollis

I am trying to recall times when the illness brought feelings of shame.

When I am doubled over with unexpected pain, I experience elements of vulnerability. But vulnerability is not always rooted in shame. Much of the shame I experienced was associated with some sense of loss, bringing with it glimpses of autumn. The fallen leaves revealing the form once known; leaves falling like tears, the gradual diminishing of former abundance as you emerge stripped bare. And although green leaves may appear again for a brief period of time, autumn will always follow as new challenges emerge and the illness resurfaces. This ongoing adaptation is a direct response to the knock-on effect the surgery brings to a system that is interconnected, a system constantly defaulting to balance despite ongoing shifts in functioning and structural changes.

So the adaptation to the losses and the rewriting of the narrative change over time. We have our backs to the wall, bare, sans former trappings, reliant solely on our inner grit in the journey ahead. Losses and transformation force you to confront who you essentially are in this one-off journey called life. Your illness becomes an invitation to embrace life again, albeit differently. And to those around you it magnifies their possible role in this journey, heightening their ability or inability to walk a road with you, their own mortality, their unfinished business and the brevity of life. The loss of you is their loss too, as they confront the fleeting moments of what we call life.

The surgery forces one to confront the realisation that the body is fragile and at this particular junction some aspect of its functioning is failing you, resulting in compromised ability to function in the world. The shame that comes with one's body failing, of feeling ill when people far older than you appear fit, feels like weakness. Feeling like the sickly animal at the back of the pack, failing to keep up, being left behind, being vulnerable and unprotected, not knowing how much longer you can keep up with the herd. And what if you get left behind and are unable to fend off the threat of failure? So yes, shame, vulnerability and fear all play a part.

This is a portrait of how I really feel:

Life is about survival, of fighting the battles, of being able to stand your ground, being self-sufficient, resilient and able to soldier on. And when you do not have the resilience or resources to ride the storm so to speak, there is a sense of shame, of vulnerability, of fear.

A huge part of it is feeling that you are out of control of your life. The change in status on many levels that illness brings with it (social isolation, financial vulnerability, inability to work owing to the unpredictability of the condition) plays into one's own sense of self. My physical decline left me largely isolated and disempowered, unable to predict my days, unable to make commitments I might not be able to honour. More than feeling alone, one is faced with the feeling of being forgotten.

The shame associated with the vulnerability and discomfort repeatedly experienced when needing to be examined is often not raised by women. When I sat opposite my surgeons and found myself describing bowel movements and consistency in detail, urinary incontinence, vaginal pain, etcetera, I cringed at the nature of the dialogue. Is this what it had all come to?

How do surgeons tolerate these graphic conversations and resultant images of voiding and excretion? Here are some of the things we do not speak of, topics shrouded in embarrassment and shame, some of which are my direct experiences, others that women in similar situations have told me:

» Do we share with them the times following surgery when uncontrolled bowel movements in the bath left one swimming in faeces?
» Do they know of the time when watery bowel movements left a trail behind you on your way to the bathroom?
» Do they know of your struggle with compaction post-surgery when with a gloved hand you tried to ease evacuation in a stitched up area of raw flesh and the excruciating pain endured as a function of the compaction?

- » Do they know of the wedging and the broken toilet seats that needed replacement?
- » Do they know of the time you stood waiting for a taxi, bottle of water in hand and suddenly realised that you had become incontinent. Thankfully, you had the good sense to spill the bottle of water over yourself to mask the puddle next to your feet!

The same applies to describing infections, and being examined; some doctors attend to you with incredible sensitivity, others leave you feeling certain that they must have been raised by wolves.

These are examples of shame. Fear-producing shame lurks in the form of incontinence, body failure, fear of embarrassing oneself, reticence of the sickly connotation of what is happening to you.

Q Do they know of any cases where the surgery had a secondary gain for patients?

There are women who have undergone pelvic floor surgery and are able to resume sexual intercourse, but seek the assurance from their gynaecologist that their husbands need not know this. This may be the secondary gain of pelvic floor surgery for some women. The surgery has given them the freedom to hang a STOP sign on an aspect of their lives they no longer want to participate in.

Q Do they know of the extent of the lack of sexual intimacy brought on by the surgery?

Do they know of the loss you experienced when sexual intimacy was no longer an active choice and the impact that it had on your marriage of twenty-five years standing?

Do they know how you pulled away, avoided intimacy not because you were not experiencing 'skin hunger' but because it reminded you that you were now less of a women, less desirable, no longer whole?

Do they know of your husband's heartache as he lies next to you in bed at night unable to connect in a sensually significant way, only to be pushed away by his wife, out of a feeling of brokenness and not because the love has changed? What flowed in demonstrativeness is now a memory, a *mokita*[36], that of which you do not speak, breeding avoidance and subsequent alienation in a once-intimate relationship?

Does he tell you of the fantasies and the possible indiscretions this surgery has brought in its wake, leaving you feeling robbed, compromised in your choices, lonely and disconnected from someone you loved and still love deeply?

For those women who enjoy sex and intimacy, but are robbed of it through radical surgery, the loss can be immense. They yearn for the life they lived, the ease with which they could pursue and give expression to their sexuality/intimacy coupled with the satisfaction that it brought. It is painful because it includes the loss of feminine power, prowess, a new identity not chosen and a sexual role denied. It incorporates a host of things that preclude your usual way of being in the world.

When one is recovering from major surgery, in extensive pain, struggling to accept what is happening to you, a partner's needs for intimacy aren't even a small blip on your radar. Intimacy is affected

---

36 That which everyone knows and no one speaks of; the Papuans of New Guinea judge the health of a community by the number of mokitas that exist within it

and is experienced by one's partner as rejection. It cuts to the core of your humanity, your bonds and your vows.

I felt wounded, devalued, redefined and robbed of my womanhood in the shrouded silence that ensued as I tried to come to terms with what had happened. The surgery forced me to redefine my role as a woman. This was painful for me because it was a loss that remained hidden from view. Internal suffering is more brutal because it is not sanctioned, remains unspoken and receives no comfort. The surgery brought with it adaptations that required resilience, fortitude, soul searching, grief and comfort in faith. It also required a review of what was possible and what needed to be adapted. I drew up a list of dreams that I thought were possible, and deleted them one by one.

Shortly after my third surgery, my journal entry reflects the feelings that it engendered.

> *There are men who desire; those who walk out the door*
> *Those who make love to your body, despite the odd flaw*
> *Those that caress God's creation, and savour its form*
> *Those who bring roses, and break promises by morn*
> *Those who honour commitment, those who leave in haste*
> *Those who caress form in the midnight, to avoid distaste*
> *Those who know of your journey, and honour its form*
> *Who have been there, dwelt there, and waited till dawn*
>
> *Then came the surgeries that ripped through silent screams*
> *And severed the memories of wholeness and being*
> *As it tore through my muscles and fibres and cells*
> *Which had lay dormant, silent and surfaced with howls*
> *And it left me half woman, half pleasure, half pain*
> *And awoke me in nights to the writhing in vain*

> *I am left wondering, quietly, while everything has changed*
> *If there are stories to be written or pleasures regained*
> *To set aside mourning to welcome the dawn*
> *Of new journeys to savour, new stories to take form*

Q Did women undergoing pelvic floor surgeries present with a specific profile as a function of their required surgery or was their history more telling of gender concerns rooted in their history?

I gave much thought to this concept, having been the recipient of the many narratives that women had shared with me over the years. I shall share some with you and you can draw your own conclusion.

I think that many women, but not all women, walk with shame related to their private parts, period. When a woman sits in front of a surgeon, how little does he know of the experiences in her histories rooted in her pelvic floor? He is unaware of the Pandora's box surgery may unleash. How on earth is he to assess whether a patient is at risk and in need of additional support during this trying recovery period?

What about those women whose marriages are devoid of fidelity, where women from both sides of the divide, religious and non-religious, contract sexually transmitted diseases from their husbands, often needing to resort to surgery for treatment. That is one aspect. The deep shame that HPV or other sexually transmitted diseases leave one feeling violated, unclean, betrayed.

Why must a woman navigate the corridors of shame brought on by the shameless perpetrator? What is the impact of HPV on the lives of women undergoing pelvic floor surgery when their inner organs are riddled with scar tissue from repeated infections gifted to them by soulless partners? Surgeons are left with very little healthy tissue where the mesh can be attached.

Can you imagine the rage that must surface in such a woman when her current condition and its recovery have been compromised by the indiscretions of a husband who violated her trust?

Many women, but not all women, have histories that have, for one reason or another, shamed them within their cultural context. In my infertility research on couples undergoing in vitro fertilisation, it was interesting how couples dealt with infertility when the male partner was the infertile partner. In such instances, it was not uncommon for the wife to own her husband's infertility, sparing his feelings of shame.

What happens to women who take on other people's shame? How does it affect the narrative of who they are?

How do women cope with the options they are faced with within a specific cultural context when they are the infertile partner and unable to conceive? Would they have to contend with the culture-specific choices their husbands were sanctioned to take in each instance? In some cultures, a second wife can be taken. In some, infertility is grounds for divorce, leaving the infertile woman within a context that is experienced as shameful, humiliating and imposed.

Many women, but not all women, experience feelings of not being the ideal feminine form, of lacking desirability, of missing the mark.

Many women, but not all women, experience shame-based experiences related to their genital area of which they do not speak. Young women in our underprivileged communities remain at home during menstruation because they are unable to afford sanitary towels. Imagine the hours lost to education, the disadvantage experienced by young girls, the 'shame' of their inability to attend to their menstruating needs because of abject poverty. How are they left feeling as women?

At a seminar I attended, an eleven-year-old child from the Cape Flats spoke of how she walked to and from school each day. On the way gang members would lie in wait for these innocent young girls and rape them, sometimes gang-rape them. She was only eleven, but had experienced more than a dozen rapes. What message about her worth rooted in her pelvic area does a child who experiences this violation feel? Imagine the feeling of violation, of shame, of being unbearably defenceless. Imagine years hence, she is your patient about to undergo pelvic floor surgery. What images and memories lie stored in her unconscious that genital surgery undertaken by a male surgeon will expose?

These are the untold stories that women walk with – stories of violation, intrusion, debasement, rape. Statistics bear out that one in four women will be physically violated in her lifetime. One of these four women may be your mother, your sister, your aunt, your daughter, your granddaughter, your cousin, your partner, your lover, your friend, your daughter-in-law, or any combination of these.

There are two kinds of secrets: those we hide from others and those that we hide from ourselves. Whichever adaptation we default to, nothing leaves us more lonely and vulnerable than our secrets. The secrets of which we do not speak eat away at our soul, leaving destruction in their wake. We do not speak because our contexts do not allow us to speak our truth, and there is an overwhelming fear that if we do, we will not be deserving of love and belonging.

Female genital surgery leaves a woman feeling vulnerable, exposed, often compromised. From between those legs and the space of that womb, emanate the stories of deep pain embedded in their histories, silenced by shame, unspoken of, but exposed through an innocent and well-meaning act of surgery. Within these withheld narratives, lies deep shame and voiceless grief, all serving to compromise the healing journey. These are the untold stories that make this journey difficult for women.

Q What role did forgiveness play in the journey of recovery?

I thought about this for a long time. First and foremost, I had to forgive myself for not knowing what I didn't know before I learnt it. I had to forgive myself for:

» allowing myself to be disempowered by another's action,
» being unable to love and forgive myself or to love and forgive others,
» the self-destructive hold I allowed the wounding to have in my life,
» not being able to return to my roots,
» turning my back on community.

Despite all this, I am grateful for the insights, the struggle, the transformative process and the ability to see a sliver of the dawn. I am grateful that I can engage in this dance of life with different steps, to a different rhythm, with different words. I am grateful for the many lessons the wounding taught me:

» to suspend judgement
» to validate experiences
» to choose my battles wisely
» to appreciate the Divine order in my life
» to see the beauty in suffering
» to embark on a spiritual quest

…to name a few.

I journaled these wounds in the safest place I knew, my sanctuary, and only in time was I able to take it to another sanctuary to be listened to, heard and witnessed. Such was my shame experienced by the child within and carried within me all these years. I am almost certain that there are no instances where I would want to reconcile with those who perpetrated the wounding, precisely because the element of trust has been forever broken and the element of betrayal remains. It is far more worthwhile in my autumn years to work on self-forgiveness based on honest reflection of who I have been, who I am at this juncture and who I am becoming in my life.

And so I conclude that illness is a metaphor, one far more complex and magnificent than I could ever have envisaged.

The challenges that illness brought in its wake and shared vignettes

On completion of the book, I was fully aware that something was lacking. The real struggle with the illness had not been given its due. What was the inner dialogue that allowed me to keep a large slice of my truth from the narrative? In a sense, my own shame related to pelvic floor prolapse and the journey that accompanied it was too difficult to share. What then was the purpose of the book? Had my shame enlisted me into the conspiracy of silence of which I accused others? The truthful answer is yes.

I wondered who I was protecting through this silence. There were many unspoken truths related to this journey that I was forced to express when my editor, in her wisdom, decided to pose questions to elicit answers that would shed light on the inner journey, the unspoken fears, the main challenges and the myths that I had to encounter.

Then I came across the works of Brigitte Jordan, an anthropologist. She had written a book titled *Birth in Four Cultures* in which she compared birthing systems according to what she calls authoritative knowledge. According to her definition, various knowledge systems (doctors, nurses, specialists) in a specific shared context (hospital) explain the way things are in the world according to their own framework. In a hospital setting, the dominant knowledge system is medical, so it carries the most weight (efficacy) and power (structural superiority), or both. She views healthcare providers' biomedical knowledge as the underlying reason why they are able to make justified decisions on patient care given their medical knowledge. This does not mean that the diagnosis they make is necessarily the correct one. The knowledge of which she speaks is simply acknowledged in this specific medical setting and community as "legitimate, consequential, worthy of discussion, and appropriate for justifying particular actions." This stance adopted by healthcare providers by definition devalues the experiences of the very patients whom they serve.

Within this framework, Jordan researched women experiencing pelvic organ prolapse. She acknowledges that these women had neither the medical terminology and/or language with which to express their subjective concerns and experiences. She attributes the dearth of narratives by women in this area as evidence of that. I would argue that this may be one aspect, but then there are also many others, shame being one of them.

Jordan identified three themes in her study. She noted that the authoritative knowledge is held by the healthcare provider and is considered legitimate by all participants. Secondly, both the women and the doctors valued the authoritative knowledge of the doctors over their own personal experience of the illness. Thirdly, the women described how they attempted to gain authoritative knowledge related to their particular illness, in order to discuss their concerns. In a sense, the subjective reality of the patient in experience of their illness is negated by the medical profession.

I began to wonder why I had allowed myself to be subjected to the same experience. It became clear to me how overwhelmed I had felt undergoing these treatments with a diminished medical background, a non-existent authoritative knowledge base and how this influenced our dialogues. To be truthful, I felt overwhelmed by all the information. It was only when I put pen to paper that clarity slowly crept in. I realised that I had colluded with this authoritative knowledge, but that my own experience was far more on target in terms of my well-being than the answers trotted out by medical personnel. I shall share some examples with you.

I began to toy with the various 'facts' that I had entertained while undergoing treatment that were not only erroneous, they were downright inaccurate, but spoken from an authoritative knowledge base I had foolishly acted upon.

Fiction #1: You can return to work within four weeks.

Really? Six hours in surgery with an abdominal scar from your chest bone to the pubic hairline, held together with sutures and steel clamps. You wake up to morphine pumps to keep you pain-free, a bed that you can adjust to make yourself comfortable and nursing staff at your beck and call for the duration of your stay in hospital. Any and all anxieties can be addressed on the ward and reassurance provided regarding your recovery. This is not recovery. This is the week before you begin to commence with the journey of recovery and healing.

Five days later you return home to a normal bed that does not allow for your preferred position for optimal comfort. Then there is severely compromised stomach and core muscle tone post-surgery, a stapled-up belly, increased pain as you attempt to become mobile, coupled with negligible understanding of what to expect in terms of recovery. And if my experience was anything to go by, I had never met anyone who had undergone pelvic floor surgery before.

So you painstakingly hold onto the railings at the back your bed to move yourself from one side to another and surround yourself with cushions to minimize post-operative pain.

Believe me when I tell you that you do not feel well, as you commence navigating this uncharted territory. By the four-week mark, you may be recovering, but you are most certainly not in a state to return to work. I would advocate that a period of three months should be allocated for recovery before returning to full-time employment and then only on advice based on each patient's unique recovery journey.

Fiction #2: Eat sensibly and body function will return to normal

Sure. You go home and are prescribed liquid drinks as you start off on foods that are easily digestible. And the hours become days and the days slowly turn into a week and still your body functioning has not returned. The word 'anxiety' comes to mind. It is that feeling of foreboding that grips you as labour sets in prior to the birthing of your first child. You cannot for the life of you imagine how you are going to give birth to something the size of a watermelon. What would you call this? Being unrealistic? Frightened? I mean, a whole watermelon. How about terrified?

Let's not forget that this is the first time that you have undergone surgery of this nature. There is no reference point. No heroine who survived the first bowel movement with a smile on her face as faeces works its way past newly inserted sutures holding raw flesh together.

The only advice you are given is "Do not strain" and "Do not become compacted."

Now, you tell me, who in their right mind would choose either option when confronted with this situation? And as the hours tick by, you realise that you are compacted and that straining would have no impact either way. And when doubled over in pain, you request an admission to hospital, but it is declined in exchange for a sachet of Precopep.

You resort to waiting. Three days go by, and by now you are close to two weeks of compaction in a stitched-up, stapled abdomen. In total desperation, you resort to a bath of boiling water hoping to dislodge the compaction manually. An hour later you are screaming uncontrollably with pain as the compaction dislodges and your partner is left to assist you in ways unimaginable, devoid of any dignity, as you are washed down, slipped into the next clean disposable nappy and returned to bed exhausted to fall asleep. But not for long.

Fiction #3: Based on my medical experience…

Based on *what* experience? Oh, you must be referring to your authoritative knowledge!

Four hours go by and you wake up needing to urinate. All you need to do is find the strength to rise from the bed, slowly work your way to the toilet, sit down, pee, the usual honours and then back to bed. Normally this can be done within 30 seconds. But that was then and this is now.

So what the hell happened between the recognition of the need to pee and the missionary position you find yourself in on the bathroom floor? You are woken up by someone screaming, only to realise that it is you. You have passed out and are now coming round, unable to move at all, having hurt your back during the fall.

Once again, an ambulance arrives to readmit you to hospital in the wee (excuse the pun) hours of the morning. I spend five days in hospital. I receive physiotherapy twice a day and tell the doctors that I have a bladder infection. They reassure me that I do not have one. I tell them that this is not possible. They tell me the test results are negative. This is day five, I'm pissed off (again, excuse the pun) and about to be discharged because I am regarded as well.

I am 60 years old for G-d's sake. Surely I should know by now what a bladder infection feels like. Enraged, I give them that silent stare, then daringly and unashamedly I remove a pad from between my legs under the sheet, covered in pus, and say, "Are you telling me I am not infected?" Within an hour, I am put on high doses of antibiotics and the attending surgeon apologises for the error, reminding me that doctors should always listen to their patients. You got that right, I think.

And so I am discharged. A few mornings later, I rise for breakfast. Feeling dizzy, I excuse myself from the table and lie down. Within 30 minutes, I am shivering, sweating and beginning to lose consciousness. Crying, I ask for help. "Please get me to the hospital." The surgeon informs me that I can only be admitted if my general practitioner deems this necessary! My friend drives me to my general practitioner's practice. He takes one look at me and calls for an immediate admission. All this in the space of four weeks.

Fiction #4: There is no biological basis for the pain levels you are describing

Subtext: I think this calls for a referral to a psychiatrist.

I begin waking at night to something I can only describe as 'nerve pain'. It feels like your body has been severely sunburnt and someone is brushing your skin with a carpet brush. The shooting pain travels in all directions, on pathways never before discovered. It is all-consuming and overwhelming. Every move you make exacerbates the pain. When I describe the nature of the pain, I know it does not exist for them because it isn't listed in the current DSM 5 under "Chronic pelvic pain associated with bristle brush."

I am diagnosed with Chronic Pelvic Pain Syndrome. But I have a tender to honour and need to return to work. No problem, up the pain medication dosages and you can pull it off. I am prescribed a cocktail of Lyrica, Prozac, Trepaline[37] and Molipaxin[38] for pain relief. Oh, forgot to mention the existing chronic medication and their possible interactions.

Fiction #5: Surgery cannot cure this presenting problem
Subtext: There is nothing more that surgery can address

In 2016 I would wake up at nights crying, feeling as though I was giving birth, my hands grabbing for opiates to ease the pain. Waking up crying became something I got used to, as I did to the realisation that something serious was wrong in my body.

Biofeedback from the physiotherapist served only to exacerbate the pain. An hour to two of therapy would have me take to my bed for two to three days. This is not normal in anybody's books. But when a surgeon tells you that this is the treatment that you need, the physiotherapist assures you that this is normal, and you are committed to getting well, there doesn't seem to be much choice, but to continue to genuflect at the altar of authoritative knowledge. All three have the same goal.

Fiction #6: Others do not go through this

More than once I was told that other patients did not respond this way. What exactly is the subtext of such a comment? Well, the subtext from someone in the medical profession who deals with authoritative knowledge is that they know, as a matter of fact, that there is nothing tangible that could be causing this level of distress.

37 A tricyclic anti-depressant used for some chronic nerve pain
38 A tricyclic anti-depressant also used for some chronic nerve pain

Now, assuming that there is nothing wrong with the patient, where does this leave the patient? Logically she would need to entertain the possibility that she is a hypochondriac of note. But whose reality is more valid – the surgeon with authoritative knowledge or the patient who has lived in her body for some 63 years? Think about that question for a while.

Q You have and still do undergo a great deal of pain. How does pain distort your reality?

Small things really.

Momentary respites: I will be watching television and become aware that I feel so at peace and am smiling and it has nothing to do with what I am watching. It has to do with the realisation that in that moment that I am not in pain. These are magical moments, ones I cherish.

Windows of the soul: Looking at my eyes in the mirror, mostly they look glazed and narrowed as if looking into the sun. Eyes are the gateway to the soul. Pain clouds the light to this gateway. Without pain killers, I look numb, like someone suffering from grief. Then I take painkillers and an hour later I return to the mirror and now my eyes are dancing, sparkling and I smile at my happy reflection, knowing full well that it took a little help from my friends to reach this point that reminds me of who I used to be.

Unreliable there-ness: A friend will phone to say they want to visit me. They arrive and I am happy to see them. Then I realise that I need to go to the toilet and excuse myself for a moment. I have a brief bowel action with ease and return to the room. But something has changed in an instant. I feel nauseous, I am white in the face and the debilitating pain is suddenly there full force. I grab for painkillers, apologise and make my way to bed where I go foetal until the medication kicks in and I can sleep off the pain. My friends know to just lock up, throw the key back into my apartment and that we will talk a little later when I am back to normal.

Momentary overload: I will be sitting in company, relaxed and chatting and find myself having to cope with rising pain. It happens rather quickly and in no time, I am aware that I'm withdrawing from the context, becoming irritable and unable to cope with the external context and its associated noise. The patience I had five minutes ago has disappeared into the ether as my attention is sapped away by the pain. I find this ongoing break with my reality inconvenient and embarrassing.

Unable to honour appointments: I promise to come for supper or go on an outing and cannot assure you whether in fact I will be able to honour it.

Sudden onset: I am sitting in the lounge working on my book, wedged 45 degrees into the arm of the couch as sitting upright is too painful. I feel well, the creative juices are flowing. It is a form of high. Then I realise that I am thirsty and think to make myself a cup of tea. I rise and am overcome with pain I did not know was there and am barely able to make it to the kitchen. In one second, I am literally catapulted into a feeling of being ill in contrast to the sense of wellness I experienced only seconds before.

The false self in the external world: I never exit my home if I am not feeling well. I only exit when I feel good and so the 'me' that people encounter looks happy and well. But if they were to see me an hour later or had seen me an hour earlier, they would not believe it is the same person. Only those who know me well are able to pick up the subtle shifts that speak of imminent change. For the rest, I am simply doing remarkably well, possibly even malingering.

Q Give me a before-and-after comparison between the 'healthy' you six months to a year prior to surgery and who you are now in terms of bodily functioning and mental focus.

You are forced to question bodily signals previously clear and distinct. It is almost like learning a different body language.

Then: You are sitting on your bed at night reading a book and need to go to the toilet. Off you toddle, do what needs to be done, do all the necessary honours, and return to bed.

Now: You are sitting on your bed and experience a feeling of needing to bear down. You need to go to the toilet … or do you? Is this a feeling that will produce something 15 hours from now or do you need to go to the toilet right now?

You go to the bathroom and seat yourself, but the connection between the lower extremities of your body and your mind has long disappeared. The alarm was false. Or maybe you are becoming compacted again? You experience yourself peeing and smile at how normally this happens. Then you realise that you have peed on the floor because the urine is now exiting sideways for some reason only known to the powers that be. In utter amazement and horror, you look on at this mess and realise that when you blamed your grandson for peeing on the floor, it was absolutely unfounded.

Then you feel like you need to defaecate. You wedge and when done you stand up like a two-year-old to view the production first hand. Much like you did when you were a child in awe of the fact that you had a body that was working, that produced something that means that it is healthy and more importantly made everyone else happy, judging by their smiles. But what you see bears no relation to what you experience. The two do not connect. You can feel that you have had a movement, but in fact see nothing in the bowel. Then you feel anxious. Another cycle, another one of those days, you think. You do the honours, wash down the toilet and the floor, meticulously cleaning everything. What was once a five second procedure now takes on a life of its own. Do I share this with my doctor? No. Do I share it with the physiotherapist? No. Why not? Shame.

Previously I would return to my work happy as a lark. Now the downward pressure has kicked in a pain cycle. You feel that something is pressing on a pain point. How does one alleviate this? Should I use a suppository to assist me? But you know that although this might help, it will bring on a new pain cycle with debilitating ramifications for the rest of the day. Something so simple and so complex runs and ruins your quality of life.

These are the secrets of which we do not speak. The behind-closed-doors suffering we spare you. The sheer shame of our incapacity.

Q How has your body changed over the last year?

I sit back in the cold light of day wondering what the catalyst will be for the next stage of regression in the illness. For example, following my third surgery I thought everything would be fine, but the surgery lasted three months before symptoms reappeared.

I went to see a Professor of Gynaecology. The rectocele had collapsed and needed repair. The surgery ensued and was declared a success. Eight weeks later I presented with incontinence and a fifth surgery followed. Now I wait for the next progression in the illness and wonder when this will require an intervention. And I honestly wonder how much more of this my body can take, let alone my psyche. What if I choose not to intervene? How will it all end?

I thought the enterocele would be the next presenting problem. But no, I am now unable to function optimally resulting in full-blown large intestinal blockage, which leaves me unbelievably distended and in chronic pain. I cannot sleep. I am nauseous. I am vomiting and experiencing excessive reflux and constantly gagging. None of my clothes fit me because I am so distended. I seek out the help of a gynaecologist because I am about to embark on a flight abroad. X-rays reveal a full large intestinal blockage. That night is a night from hell. By 7.00 am I am sitting opposite my doctor. He contacts the surgeon who performed the first three surgeries and has me admitted to hospital for faecal flushing. The compaction is extensive. Conservative options won't correct this. This is impending perforation. I hate to think what could have happened if I had undertaken the flight without appropriate intervention.

My children have paid for my ticket to holiday with them in Israel. I do not want to be a party pooper, so am imbibing 8 to 10 Tramacet[39] a day trying to mask the pain in order to keep up with the programme. But after day four, my body goes on strike and debilitated with pain I resort to bed for days until balance is achieved once again and I am able to repeat the pattern. Get with the programme, take the tabbies, become compacted, resort to bed, do what needs to be done, achieve homeostasis and return to life once again to repeat the cycle… And this is called life.

While in Israel, I developed a persistent cough, which continued for four months. In early 2017, a gastroscopy revealed a hiatus hernia[40] and the diagnosis of GERD[41].

Some six weeks later, a second umbilical hernia[42] was diagnosed, which had been brought on by increased bearing down during

39 An opiate painkiller

40 Protrusion of the stomach through the oesophageal opening in the diaphragm

41 Gastro-oesophageal Reflux Disease

42 Part of the intestine protrudes through the umbilical opening in the abdominal muscles

evacuation. Soon thereafter, structural narrowing of the anal canal made evacuation virtually impossible. With the aid of laxatives, body functioning continued, but this was not a solution to a serious problem. With no ability to bear down, a near-closed anal canal, and two additional hernias, talk of a colostomy surfaced.

Q What do you tell yourself in moments of despair, humiliation and fear?

I tell myself to finish the book so that I can leave something behind that will break the silence and will prove that despite being brought to my knees, my commitment to life remained. I could still make a contribution despite the illness. My life has purpose despite the illness. I have conquered the illness in the short term despite the challenges. My bodily functioning is compromised, some days more than others, but definitely regressing overall.

So I think to myself, how much longer before my quality of life becomes so compromised that another surgery is required. Then I ask myself, what is the purpose of all the surgeries if the window period is becoming smaller and smaller. I don't foresee a normal life expectancy. I have just attended my granddaughter's bat mitzvah. If I am blessed, maybe in two years' time I can attend my grandson's bar mitzvah.

But I have no long-term plans. Those I have deleted. I live in the moment and for the moment with very realistic consideration given to the way forward. My grandchildren speak openly of what they see and whether I will be at their next celebration or a wedding. Then they look at me and ask me to send them a symbol so that they know that if I am no longer with them, they can know that I am there in spirit. These are not dialogues I shun. They are gifts in a way.

In moments of despair I surrender to G-d. I have little to no control to stall or circumvent this progression. There is no fear. I have stopped worrying. It serves no point. Just trust in the process and in compassion. What more is there one can do? I am a player in this cosmic drama and everything will unfold exactly as it should.

Q If you could have anything in the world, what would it be?

I have most things I need. I am truly blessed. I see my children and grandchildren, which many people are deprived of owing to immigration or as a result of the shrapnel of relationships. I believe that I have achieved much of what I was meant to in this lifetime.

There is little unfinished business at this point. Those that I would have entertained are not essential to the journey.

I would have liked a relationship with a man of substance, but do not foresee this. I am okay with that. I have always wanted to visit the camps in Poland, but this does not feel feasible at this juncture. I would love to experience less stress around financial concerns related to the long-term cost of the illness on my quality of life. But not much else. I am reconciled to life as it has unfolded. I think the important work, the inner journey, has for the most part been achieved.

I am not sure I can say the same of my spiritual journey, despite leading a deeply spiritual and considered life. There are relationships that have devolved into puddles that have been extremely disappointing, but I realise their inherent limitations.

I fear indignity, of living life on other people's terms, of decisions being made about my life over which I have no control. This is what I struggle with because it feels as though the human component is missing and the practical component takes precedence. I think what I would have appreciated beyond all else would have been a loving holding environment to hold me in my frailty with dignity.

What would I like most in all in the world? A family, a life filled with meaning, my health, my faith, good friends, shelves of books, good music, chilled glasses of wine, sunsets, warm fire places, much laughter, stories to tell. And above all, to be surrounded by opportunities to love and be loved. Therein lies the secret.

Q What was the most traumatic incident in your entire journey?

There is nothing more soul destroying than being in experience of a health crisis and being told that it is all in your head, or having the symptoms being brushed aside entirely, or being put on a conveyer belt to nowhere with inappropriate referrals and stalled intervention because of the view that the patient is not ill.

Q Why is it that a woman's experiences or self-concept of her condition are devalued and/or ignored?

The collusion to silence pelvic organ prolapse is partly protective. The medical fraternity would not be able to deal with the onslaught of women seeking healthcare solutions to bodily symptoms that they have not been educated about.

When I wanted to read for a doctorate in this field, I was quite shocked when asked by a researcher what I would do if I came across concerns around patient care that would compromise the surgeons involved. I was taken aback by this. My motive for doing the research was to allow for an in-depth experience of women's stories to come to light. In passing, the researcher said that many incidences have come to the fore where the patients were less than satisfied with the outcome of received treatment.

There is a lack of accountability and transparency around treatment, and service evaluation of patients is not encouraged. At what cost do women then keep silent?

Jordon's small research study confirmed that the bio-medical knowledge is considered authoritative over women's experiential knowledge. While she entertains the possibility of "equally legitimate, parallel knowledge systems…where people move easily between them," she grapples with the concern of how this can be achieved in the minefield of pelvic organ prolapse.

She stresses that it is important to note the language women use to describe pelvic organ prolapse. This sets the basis for shared understanding, transcending the need for authoritative knowledge. Women often struggle to describe the symptoms they experience. This highlights the need to listen to the spoken and unspoken interactions between these women and their attending healthcare practitioner.

Special attention needs to be paid to either under-diagnosing or over-diagnosing any presenting condition. This stance negates women's experience in a health crisis already shrouded in silence. Negation of one's reality is a shaming and deeply disturbing experience. We need to give women a voice for their health concerns through languaging it in words familiar to them, nuances and all, to avoid hiding the substance of their experience in clinical terms. More attention needs to be paid to women's descriptions of their current physical symptoms.

This brings me to an evaluation of the entire experience and gratitude for the things I've learnt since the illness began, and am still learning.

CHAPTER FIVE

THE THINGS ILLNESS TAUGHT ME

By the six-year mark, I had gained a better understanding of what caused illness and, more specifically, what ensured healing, and I came to the following conclusion, expressed in a quote by Rebecca Beard:

> *The cause is within us. The cure is within us. When we know this, our concept of disease is no longer that of something fixed upon the body cells which must be purged, cut or burned away. It is not something coming in from the outside which we cannot prevent. Rather, it is a change from within, and we must find the reason why the body changes its perfect pattern to vibrate to discord rather than to harmony.*

The gift of time and changed perceptions

According to James Hollis, in the second half of life, the questions become: "Who, apart from the roles you play, are you? What does the soul ask of you? Do you have the wherewithal to shift course, to deconstruct your painfully achieved identity, risking failure, marginalization and loss of collective approval?" No small task.

This resonated for me during this time out of time and forced me to grapple with many existential realities, while confronting numerous changes and seeking adaptations to them. Most certainly the illness complicated the questions that arose and demanded different answers as well as different paths. In retrospect, I view this as a gift of great magnitude, forcing me on a healing path of a different nature.

Our ability to see the wonder of the world that surrounds us allows us to elevate the familiar to the sacred. Once we are able to see the world in what Rabbi Abraham Joshua Herschel calls *radical amazement*, we are truly able to appreciate all of creation, each contact, the significance of each life, even the very familiar.

The fact that the sun rises every day and that we are able to awake each morning bears testimony to G-d's faithfulness to return our souls to us. Our souls are returned to us each day because we have not completed that which G-d has sent us to do. The lived experience bears testimony that we are playing a part in the design that G-d has for our lives, often unaware of how short that would be.

So we are given the gift of time. We are often lulled into a sense of complacency believing naively that there will always be a tomorrow. Often we ignore the possibility that a greeting, a smile, or a harsh word may indeed come to signify the last memory that we have of a person. It is indeed difficult to live life with the intensity that this level of awareness would require of us.

And so the illness brought home to me through my daily prayer rituals the gratitude I had for surviving the illness thus far. The prayer that is recited on rising each morning took on new significance during this time:

> *I thank You, G-d, Eternal One,*
> *for lovingly restoring my soul to me,*
> *filled with Your eternal trust.*

The gift of living in awe of G-d's creation

When we are not ill we take almost everything for granted. But when our bodily functions begin to fail us, the wonder of the intricacies of the human body gain new perspective. And so it was that I whispered the 'after-bathroom' blessing known as Asher Yatzar[43] with a new intensity many times during the day.

> *Blessed are You, Hashem, our G-d, King of the universe,*
> *who formed man with wisdom and created within him many openings and hollows. It is revealed and known before the Throne of Your glory*
> *That if one of them were to be closed or if one of them were to be opened,*
> *it would be impossible to survive even for a brief time.*
> *Blessed are You, Hashem, Who heals all flesh and acts wondrously.*

The gift of comparisons between the old life and the new

Surrendering to the polarities of life forces one to balance one's views and explore one's illness and its impact more fully. We need to normalise our view of illness because, in a sense, it is a marker for where the shifts have taken place, both internal and external. Here are some examples of the comparisons with which I grappled:

---

43 Who formed

- The life I lived would be the catalyst for a life in review
- The feeling of impending death heralded an impending rebirth
- Where there was darkness, light would return
- Rather than planning a life, I could plan a life after the illness
- Past independence would be replaced with modified independence
- My ignorance around pelvic floor would be replaced by knowledge
- From initial feelings sprang hope and transformation
- From feelings of abandonment arose feelings of support
- From living through ego I could now live through Divine grace
- Illness was the catalyst for a new commitment to health and to life
- My need to be in control was replaced by my surrender to forces greater than myself

The gift of purpose

My illness was an invitation to my purpose. It taught me the importance of narrative based on my lived experience. To teach, you have to have a grasp of the concepts you wish to impart to others. And what better way to learn than through lived experience?

My illness called for a re-evaluation of my values, beliefs and modus operandi in the world. I had to explore many aspects of my being. So I think through some finger of fate or faith, I began to realise that despite the fact that my body was failing me, it did not detract from me and my worth. They were two different processes.

I never felt flawed because of the illness. Rather the illness made me explore avenues that were flawed. I needed to write a book to serve as evidence of a journey explored, evidence of living a considered life. I realised that dying from my illness was an active choice. And that I was not ready to die.

The gift of choosing your legacy

Despite early wounding, we can still survive the furnace. You can always change your legacy if you choose to do so consciously. So it was my choice to be a different kind of mother than the mothering I had received as a child. I had lived in the abyss, in a less-than-optimal holding environment and vowed that my children would never experience that abyss. They always had a mother to turn to, to talk to, to laugh with, to discuss their spiritual path and to guide them.

My decision at an early age not to be like my mother and to live my life despite all the deprivation was vindication enough. While my mother always told me that I would amount to nothing, I can only say, you have no idea how tall I stood on your shoulders. You were probably the catalyst for my magnificence. I thank you for the part you played unconsciously in my development and that I had the strength and wisdom to learn from it. For this, I will be forever grateful to you.

I am also grateful to you that you walked a spiritual path, a value I hold dear. You served out your contract for my growth, but I still find it difficult to think lovingly of you and I don't know if I will ever be able to pardon you. For this I am too small and too hurt. The wound has not yet healed.

I realised that there were certain actions or people which I could forgive more easily than others. I also realised that there were certain aspects of my lived experience that had caused me so much suffering that I was not yet able to forgive. So there is still work to be done.

The gift of exploring dis-ease within the body

When the soul's journey is off track, when patterns keep recurring, then it is time to attend to the unconscious. Whatever the cause of the wounding for which illness is the metaphor, what it asks of us is to heal the wounding that caused the illness in the first place. So be sensitive to the whispers of the inner landscape of your body if you wish to anticipate and participate in the dance of healing. I think that Carl Jung was right when he said that the gods visited us through illness.

A sad soul can kill us far more quickly than an illness. The challenge is to pay specific attention to all forms of dis-ease within the body. In doing so, we can benefit emotionally, mentally and spiritually. True healing implies a new relationship with oneself. Responding to this call in the depth of the night is a choice to undertake a healing journey.

You must choose to take responsibility for your healing in every sense of the word, no matter how long that journey, no matter how many obstacles along the way. It requires commitment and passion to search for a better life. You must name the demon confronting you and take on the challenge with all your being, precisely because no other person can undertake on this challenge for you.

> *If you think you are too small to make a difference, try sleeping with a mosquito.*
>
> Dalai Lama

The gift of healing and faith

Who does one turn to in times of experienced or perceived onslaught when the stressors are both internal and systemic? Usually, we would turn to organised religion, community and family structures. However, as these crumble we are left feeling alienated and unable to hear the deafening cries of disconnect. If the umbilical cord connecting G-d and man is viewed as faith, then this cord is the thinnest of threads.

The soul of man has remained locked in infancy, adrift in an ocean of feelings of estrangement from G-d. We master skills, become experts in our chosen field, and think we have arrived. There's no more work to do. And so we drift aimlessly, not knowing which questions to ask to commence the journey that will narrow the gap between the creation and the Creator. The good news is that there is no better opportunity to know G-d than when we are in this perceived abyss. Without my personal faith, this journey would not be possible, as is evident in my journal entry below:

> *Faith.*
> *How did He respond? you may ask.*
> *With what did He respond? you may ask.*
> *And I will tell you that I was given everything I needed to heal: the right healer at the right time; the strongest friends and family whose strength, support and love carried me on their wings when the flight seemed too long; sacred shelters to heal and rest my weary body; support in unimaginable ways; and perfect timing of the arrival of support that was synchronistic and magical.*

It also taught me about the charlatans and the men of straw; about those who walked their talk and those who were fake; family with heart and family devoid of soul; those you could count on and those from whom you needed to flee; and those you wanted near you and those who made you want to run into the hills.

The audit was immense but the gains plentiful. But when completed and the signature signed, I realised that I was richer than when the audit started, and I had won the battles on all fronts. My soul had met the challenge, my faith had met my Maker, my spirit had soared to meet its match and my psyche has healed to a still small point, sans despair, sans anguish, sans naming, blaming and shaming. I have just accepted that it is what it is, and it has become what it has become.

The gift of review and reframe

It is a gruesome and relentless task that illness invites us to perform. To confront our demons and frailty, and illusions about the life we have lived. To look on at the world with more compassion, gratitude, humility and hope. And I asked myself in the dead of night why the suffering continues.

» How does it serve me?
» If I were to relinquish the suffering, which new adaptations would be called for?
» What new narrative would I need to write?
» What am I hiding from?
» Which majestic self am I too afraid to own?

Deep down many of us feel very ordinary. It's the feeling of not being good enough, of not living a spectacular enough life and of not being worthy of validation for the work we've done. We spend so much of our psychic energy trying to be lovable, perfect and desirable.

Oh, the compromises we make as women, and on so many levels, when we strive to be the perfect other. We will sell our bodies before we sell our souls. We will leave our form naked, rather than share our secrets. Such is our shame. So how do we deal with this sense of inadequacy and imperfection, this sense of not being worthy enough?

We strive for perfection, hoping in desperation that this will quell our feelings of shame, lack of acceptance, rejection and betrayal. But it is only once we shame and betray ourselves that we are left with ashes in our mouths, nothing in our hands and no authentic love to show for it. This is a form of soul suffering because we are so disconnected from our inner worth, so lacking in appreciation of who we essentially are. These feelings of imperfection and vulnerability force us to face the demons that have kept us small.

> *[Daring greatly] means the courage to be vulnerable. It means to show up and be seen. To ask for what you need. To talk about how you're feeling. To have the hard conversations.*
>
> Brené Brown

A journal entry reflects my thinking:

> *Thank you, G-d, for the courage it took to wake up to life's challenge:*
> *for being brave enough to confront life head on*
> *for being able to own, explore and share my personal story*
> *for burying the old and erecting the new*
> *for only being betrayed, but not broken*
> *for the transformative experience that taught me courage*
> *for the long journey that taught me patience*
> *to face the long-avoided wounds;*
> *to face uncertainty*
> *for the ability to change outdated perceptions*
> *to go it alone;*
> *to give it voice;*
> *to be human.*
> *I thank you G-d.*

The gift of choosing your battles and your attitude

This reminds me of the story about the Cherokee.

One evening an old Cherokee told his grandson about a battle that goes on inside every person. He said, "My son, the battle is between two wolves inside all of us. One wolf is Evil. It is anger, envy, greed, arrogance, self-pity, guilt, resentment, lies, superiority and ego. The other wolf is Good. It is joy, love, hope, humility, kindness, empathy, generosity, truth, compassion and faith.

The grandson thought about it a minute and then asked his grandfather, "Which wolf wins?" The grandfather replied: "The one you feed."

Q What would you say to those who may criticise this work?

Once you have the courage to publish your writings, it goes without saying that there will be a multitude of responses. I would listen to the critics who have been in the arena, who have lived the struggle and survived none the less. Only when you have been in the arena and survived despite, is your opinion worthy of noting, even if the experience is vastly different. This book reflects the healing process that took place on a multitude of levels in response to the time out that illness demanded of me. It was my story, a human story reflecting my truth, my wounding and my healing.

Theodore Roosevelt's sentiments sum it up with precision.

> *It is not the critic who counts; not the man who points out how the strong man stumbles, or where the doer of deeds could have done them better. The credit belongs to the man who is actually in the arena, whose face is marred by dust and sweat and blood; who strives valiantly; who errs, who comes short again and again,*

> *because there is no effort without error and shortcoming; but who does actually strive to do the deeds; who knows great enthusiasms, the great devotions; who spends himself in a worthy cause; who at the best knows in the end the triumph of high achievement, and who at the worst, if he fails, at least fails while daring greatly, so that his place shall never be with those cold and timid souls who neither know victory nor defeat.*

Revisiting options and gaining perspective

And so my perspective on the fallout of the illness changed over time. As options disappeared, I realised that the years of illness had taught me well and I had a range of coping strategies at my fingertips. The now edited version of my former self forced me to explore all aspects of the illness and related complications, digesting the information in bits and sometimes with difficulty.

Quality of lifestyle became increasingly associated with a narrow corridor of light and opportunity. Wherever possible I tapped into those things that I could still manage, those things that gave me a sense of control over my life. Managing my energy became a priority.

Exploring options, however limited, was something I pursued with precision. I was no fool and realised that options and choices were slowly but surely diminishing. I found positive ways to deal with my stress levels and kept up therapy to assist with the last vestiges of buoyancy I had as I confronted my ambivalence towards any further surgical interventions.

As a child aged eleven, I had looked on as my father lived with debilitating illness for seventeen years, an option I could not envisage for myself. I wanted to see the book completed, published and the silence around pelvic floor broken once and for all.

The illness has managed to derail my life plans and, in my vulnerability, I continue to work towards meaningful goals, no matter how small, believing that a goalless life is a form of living death. I spend hours writing, researching, reading and listening to music. I only hold onto relationships that are life enhancing. The adaptation is ongoing but managed with sensitivity and care. But the clarity that the evaluation has brought was comforting, insightful and clear.

Past perceptions were reframed and restored to a place within my heart that allowed for a more compassionate version of the wounding and the impact these events had on my life.

And now, seven years later I am confronting the only option remaining, a colostomy. This difficult and painful decision, filled with trepidation, shame and silence, is the catalyst for another chance, possibly even a better quality of life. Hopefully it will allow me to continue with assisting women through therapy and support groups to explore the hidden, unspoken challenges women face when confronted with pelvic floor disorders.

And lastly, to continue with research, writing and publishing. This newly defined goal and associated challenge inspires me, beckons me and demands that I meet the challenges with hope and faith.

In my forties, I became interested in the concerns facing individuals in midlife and ran spiritual groups for woman from all walks of life. Midlife is a turning point in the lives of many individuals in cultures where aging was not venerated. And so it was at this time that I came across a poem by Sam Keen which made a profound impact on me. Over the years, it has always spurred me on, provided me with hope, and a belief that things can change and transform. It invites us to engage in life's journey, no matter the scars born of struggle, bearing testimony to a life lived, savoured, considered and survived.

In Sam Keen's dream, a man walks into his bedroom, sits on the edge of his bed and says, "I have learned one important thing in life – to begin again." Keen notes that beginning again with the wisdom we have acquired from experience and discovering who we are now is central to hope

For me personally, the journey undertaken, the wounds explored, the insights gained and the resolution sought during the time of my illness have taught me about hope, the importance of beginning again and the belief in a tomorrow. What a gift to find in the throes of adversity!

> *Hope is the thing with feathers*
> *That perches in the soul,*
> *And sings the tune without the words,*
> *And never stops at all,*
> *And sweetest in the gale is heard;*
>
> *And sore must be the storm*
> *That could abash the little bird*
> *That kept so many warm.*
>
> *I've heard it in the chillest land,*
> *And on the strangest sea;*
> *Yet, never, in extremity,*
> *It asked a crumb of me.*
>
> Emily Dickinson

CHAPTER SIX

JOB, STRUGGLE, FAITH AND MEANING

My book was born of struggle during a time of illness. In this final chapter I return to the role of faith in understanding of the purpose of my journey.

The Book of Job, one of the Wisdom books of the Bible, is highly acclaimed in literary circles. Victor Hugo noted that, "Tomorrow, if all literature was to be destroyed and it was left to me to retain one work only, I should save Job."

The Book of Job addresses the many questions that arise in the face of suffering. Why does one person thrive in adversity whereas another is wounded beyond measure? Why do righteous people suffer and the unrighteous flourish?

Job is blessed with children, immense wealth and is known as one of the greatest of all the people of the East. Satan attributes Job's righteousness to his absence of suffering, claiming his righteousness as self-serving, and if confronted by adversity, Job's faith would falter. Satan's viewpoint is that faith in the face of suffering is to be awarded greater merit than faith in the absence of suffering. G-d allows Satan to inflict suffering on Job, on the proviso that no harm will befall Job.

When G-d withdraws His Divine grace from Job, numerous systemic losses ensue. The Sabeans kill off his asses, a fire from heaven consumes his sheep, and the Chaldeans swoop down on his camels and steal them. In all instances, the young men overseeing his assets die. The final loss is brought by a great wind that collapses the four corners of Job's son's house, killing all his children, sparing only one messenger. In response to this loss, Job tears his robe, shaves his hair and falls to the ground to worship G-d, acknowledging his dependence on G-d's will for his life, believing that he has no right to question the workings of the Divine. In his grief, Job begs G-d for an explanation, but none is forthcoming.

Satan's inflicted suffering has not derailed Job's commitment to serve G-d. Displeased, Satan seeks G-d's approval to afflict Job's body with disease, rationalising that faithfulness in the absence of personal suffering is not challenging. With G-d's consent, Satan inflicts Job with boils. Experiencing pain, fever, blackened skin, rapidly declining health and fearing death, Job faces feelings of aloneness and abandonment, and believes he's been forsaken by G-d. In his anguish, he pleads with God to provide an answer as to why he has been the target of such severe suffering. With his spirit broken, awaiting his death, but his faith steadfast, G-d remains hidden and silent.

With the loss of his wealth, the news of Job's suffering reaches his fellow traders and friends, and soon Job's three friends, Eliphaz, Bildad and Zophar, join him in his period of mourning. Each in turn attempts to find the reason for Job's suffering, urging him to repent. In response, Job admonishes his friends for their harsh words and words lacking in wisdom. He holds out for a communication from G-d wherein his iniquities and sins are revealed. And finally, when G-d does respond, His counsel is brief and to the point.

> *Where wast thou when I laid the foundations of the earth? Declare, if thou hast understanding.*
> *Who hath laid the measures thereof, if thou knowest?*
> *Or who hath stretched the line upon it?*
> *Whereupon are the foundations thereof fastened?*
> *Or who laid the cornerstone thereof;*
> *When the morning stars sang together, and all the sons of G-d shouted for joy?*
>
> Job 38:1-7

Implicit in G-d's response is that He is all-knowing. Job realizes that G-d's framework is Divine, and that he is limited by his human understanding of the events. Ultimately, he comes to the realization that it is in his own hands to save himself. An understanding of the suffering does not ameliorate it precisely because it is part of the human condition. Only when Job humbles himself to G-d, accepting that he is not able to understand the workings of the Divine, and willing to forgive his friends, is he once again in receipt of God's blessings.

Illness was the catalyst for transformation, an invitation to take on a different citizenship with a different worldview born of struggle. The vulnerability that it brought in its wake was the vulnerability that comes from the disruption of the life force itself, and we are left to dance with health and illness, life and death. The unexplored suffering it unleashed allowed me to come to view illness as metaphor for unexpressed suffering. It called for a more compassionate version of my story, inviting me to decipher unconscious messages from my body most in need of acknowledgement, rectification and healing. It allowed me to address the narrative that had robbed me of becoming who I was rightfully meant to be and was becoming.

Life and the journey are processes and only when identified, lived to the full, explored without borders, will it ensure me the privilege to identify, acknowledge and reveal the gold hidden in the nugget of suffering. And so, my story continues …

In conclusion

From a relatively early age, we come to know that life is divided into stages, starting with infancy and ending with old age. We also know that each stage brings with it a change in roles. We are children of parents, then become parents ourselves. Because these stages and roles are expected, we transition through them and into them relatively easily. And even though we know there are accidents and tragedies that could befall us along the way, we are shocked when they happen.

Illness throws us off course, disrupting our expected stages of life and changes in roles. Suddenly we are in chaos and must adapt to the sick role. We and our families and friends need to adapt and live according to different rules and far different expectations. This takes resilience, courage and commitment.

If I could look the surgeon in the eye today, given the entire journey, I would thank him for being there for me all the way; for having the courage to do what needed to be done; and to tell him that he must never feel that he did not do right by me. There were too many external variables over which he had no control, to ensure a return to optimal health.

PART 2

Pelvic Organ Prolapse Guide

CHAPTER ONE

SYMPTOMS, DIAGNOSIS AND TREATMENT CHOICES

The uniqueness of each patient's experience

Every patient's narrative and surgical treatment are unique with unique outcomes. Stories about our experiences serve as a bridge between the lives of surgeons, patients and family. Each person's story will have many players and reflect many layers of the journey towards health, precisely because illness is systemic in its impact.

The women who survive the journey are those who manage to balance the highs and the lows the illness brings in its wake. Illness is the human face of clinical concerns, steeped in a dance with patients and healthcare professionals. The physical aspects of illness take their toll, while the emotional aspects can rob you of your essence. When you feel like you are treading water and not coping, be brave, reach out and ask for help. It takes great courage to ask for help when feeling vulnerable.

One thing is definite, seeking help is not weakness. Everyone needs someone to validate their experiences, to share their struggles, to feel safe and accepted. Do not allow anyone on this journey to minimise your experience or worse still, tell you that it is all psychological and in your head. This is a negation of who you are, in the body you inhabit, in experience of a health crisis.

Signs and symptoms of pelvic floor dysfunction

Women who suffer from pelvic floor syndrome can present with any number of conditions, such as:

- leaking urine during everyday activities that exert pressure on the abdomen
- difficulty urinating
- an inability to experience regular bowel movements
- constipation or other bowel problems
- discomfort or pain in the lower abdominal area
- a feeling of pressure and bloating in the abdominal area
- a lump in your vagina
- unusual bleeding or discharge
- a feeling that something is descending into the vagina
- painful intercourse
- back pain

When you begin to notice changes in the way your body feels or functions in your pelvic area, you can divide the symptoms into three categories:

- organ prolapse
- urinary incontinence
- faecal incontinence/constipation

Organ prolapse

The word 'prolapse' simply means that an organ has moved out of its natural position and is pressing on other organs. In pelvic floor prolapse, the organs that can prolapse into the vagina are the bladder, the uterus (if present), or the rectum. This happens when the supporting structures weaken over time. Muscles and connective tissue weaken when they are strained. This may happen during vaginal childbirth, chronic constipation, violent coughing and heavy lifting.

Surgery and repeated infections also cause the supporting tissue to weaken. Depending on the severity of the prolapse and how many organs are involved, this bulging can cause discomfort and even pain.

Essentially, there are five types of prolapse[44]:

- **Cystocele** occurs when the bladder bulges into the front wall of the vagina.
- **Enterocele** is when the back and front vaginal walls separate, allowing the small bowel to press against the vagina.
- **Rectocele** occurs when the back of the vagina weakens and the rectum prolapses into the vagina.
- **Uterine prolapse** occurs when the ligaments supporting the top of the vagina weaken, in turn causing other ligaments elsewhere to weaken, allowing the uterus (womb) to prolapse.
- **Vaginal vault prolapse** occurs when the upper portion of the vagina loses its normal shape and drops down. This often happens after a hysterectomy and may occur in combination with one of the other types of prolapse.
- **Urethrocele** occurs when the urethra, which transports urine from the bladder out of the body, slips and pushes against the lower part of the front of the vagina.

---

44 For more detailed information on pelvic floor prolapse, go to:
http://www.allcareforwomen.com/pelvic-floor-disorders.php
http://www.agsc.com.au/vaginal-prolapse-repair-surgery-agsc.html

Weak pelvic floor support structures most often result in urinary and faecal incontinence.

Diagram of a prolapsed pelvic floor

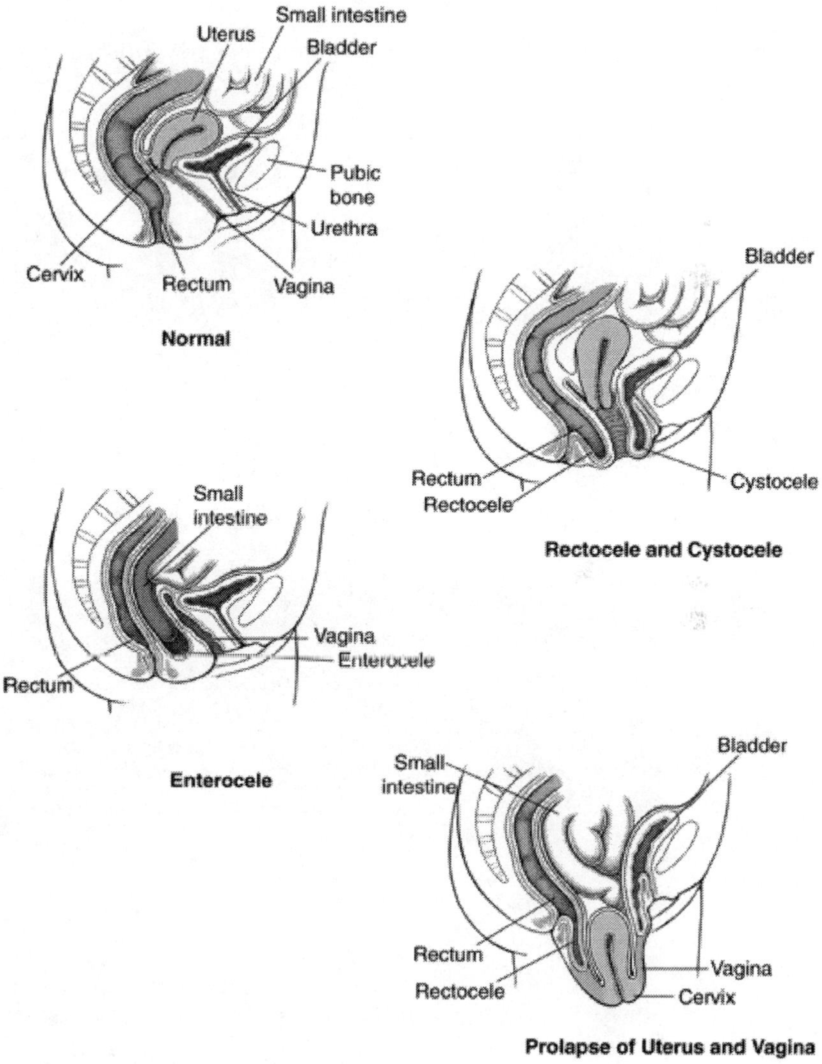

Urinary incontinence[45]

Quite simply put, urinary incontinence is loss of bladder control. This can happen when you cough or sneeze (stress incontinence), or it can be more severe in that you have a sudden urge to urinate and can't get to the toilet in time. In short, urinary incontinence is involuntary leakage of urine, something you have no control over.

Many women present with the condition during pregnancy and for those in whom it commences in later life, it is usually a function of aging and associated weakening of the pelvic floor muscles. Incontinence is not a normal condition, and the embarrassment and shame associated with this condition affects health-seeking behaviour as well as intimacy and sexuality.

Faecal incontinence[46]

Similar to urinary incontinence, faecal or bowel incontinence is an inability to control bowel movements, which results in involuntary soiling. This can be caused by weakening of the sphincter muscles that normally keep the opening of the rectum closed, a prolapsed rectum, chronic constipation or diarrhoea, or nerve damage in which signals from the rectum don't reach the brain.

In addition to chronic diarrhoea or constipation, women present with this condition as a function of aging, pelvic surgery, trauma during childbirth, obesity and other medical conditions, such as diabetes and stroke.

---

45 For more detailed information on urinary incontinence, go to: http://www.webmd.com/urinary-incontinence-oab/ss/slideshow-incontinence-in-women

46 For more detailed information on faecal incontinence, go to: http://www.webmd.com/digestive-disorders/bowel-incontinence#2-5

Do you have pelvic floor syndrome?

If you present with one or more symptoms in all three of these categories, you have pelvic floor syndrome:

PELVIC ORGAN PROLAPSE	URINARY INCONTINENCE	FAECAL INCONTINENCE
• Rectocele • Urethrocele • Enterocele • Cystocele • Uterine prolapse • Vaginal vault prolapse	• Urinary stress incontinence • Overactive bladder • 'Nervous' bladder	• Straining • Frequent bowel movements • Bloating • Abdominal pain

Knowing that you might have pelvic floor syndrome means that you can seek early diagnosis and intervention.

Menopause and gender health issues

Dealing with menopause as a rite of passage, and at the same time coping with declining health issues related to pelvic floor syndrome can be challenging because the physical and the psychological are entwined.

As women confront menopause, their sense of well-being diminishes because of decreased oestrogen. Vulva and vaginal changes may lead to dryness, painful intercourse (dyspareunia) or spotting/bleeding associated with intercourse.

Oestrogen replacement therapy can remedy or improve vaginal health and sexual functioning. While these conditions are not necessarily related to aging, it stands to reason that with women living longer, they are at higher risk of developing pelvic floor syndrome.

Diagnosis

Diagnostic tests

A routine pelvic examination would indicate further tests to be considered. These include:

- Anal manometry to evaluate the strength of the anal sphincter muscles
- Cystoscopy to view inside the bladder and urethra
- Dynamic defaecography to evaluate the pelvic floor and rectum while the patient is having a bowel movement
- Endoanal ultrasound, which uses sound waves to form a picture of the anal sphincter muscles for evaluation
- Urodynamics to evaluate bladder and urethra functioning in order to determine whether surgery is indicated

The professionals you may encounter

Choose a unit with a multi-disciplinary approach and, if possible, one that is research-based to ensure that the team is up-to-date with the latest findings in the field. The medical team are your partners on this journey. This team could consist of all or any of the following:

- Nurses, the first line of contact for patients
- Colorectal surgeons, who provide surgical treatment of the large intestine and the rectum
- Gastroenterologists, who treat the small intestine, stomach and oesophagus
- Urogynecologists, who are obstetricians/gynaecologists who specialise in the care of women with pelvic floor disorders

- Urologists, who specialise in urinary disorders in women and men
- Plastic and reconstructive surgeons
- Physical therapists
- Radiologists

Choosing the right person for the job

Choose a surgeon who is respected by colleagues, and has experience in this specific area of surgery. Find the specialist whose expertise is acknowledged, whose integrity is intact, and who is committed to healing. You must have faith in the surgeon's abilities and respect for him/her as a surgeon. This will decrease your levels of anxiety both pre- and post-operatively. Choose an approachable surgeon, one who can address intimate, complex female concerns with sensitivity, honesty and compassion.

The road from discomfort and compromised quality of life to an accurate diagnosis varies for each woman. It may involve consulting numerous specialists, however, the final diagnosis and consultation with the surgeon will determine whether the intervention will be conservative in nature or require vaginal, abdominal or laparoscopic surgery.

If you want a second opinion, this should be encouraged. If possible, involve your partner in the consultations, as this surgery will have an impact on his/her life as well.

Pre-surgical workup to pelvic organ prolapse

You may be overwhelmed by the medical jargon confronting you in this new arena. Research the topic, explore it from many angles and, above all, take responsibility for your health. The more informed you are, the more you will feel able to engage in dialogue and decisions related to treatment. Always attempt to go the conservative route first.

Remember, surgery is a structural attempt to address a complex problem. Familiarise yourself with the nature of tests required of you prior to surgery or during the workup towards a diagnosis. Request copies of all results, as these provide you with a time frame of the journey, and a transparent one at that.

Make sure that your surgeon explicitly and carefully explains your medical condition to you, preferably with diagrams or models that enable you to visualise what is happening and how the surgery will address the problem.

Make sure that you provide your doctors with a thorough medical background as well your particular psychosocial concerns. You will be asked to complete questionnaires specific to your condition. These are usually provided by the consulting surgeon to complete prior to the first consultation.

Surgical options

Available surgical options include vaginal surgery, abdominal surgery or laparoscopic surgery. Laparoscopic surgery is generally preferred because:

- the camera shows the surgeon a magnified view of the pelvic floor
- the surgeon can place stitches more precisely
- there is less bleeding
- the abdomen has not been cut open, so there is less post-operative pain and discomfort
- your hospital stay is shorter and your recovery is quicker.

The two most common operations for pelvic floor prolapse are:

» in cases of urinary incontinence, a sling procedure is done to lift and support the bladder so that the sphincter can close more easily, and
» in cases of cystocele and rectocele repairs, a sacrocolpopexy (sacral colpopexy) is performed in which a mesh is used to support the prolapsed organs.

Coping guidelines

Plan all foreseeable concerns related to your admission, surgery and discharge with military precision. Remember, your family is part of the team. Should you live alone, make sure that you have friends who can assist you in the initial stages, with chores, shopping, transport, cooking, cleaning and so on.

Avoid being isolated during the recovery period. Contact with others is healing provided they do not stay too long or don't drain you during their visits. You may want to draw up a short list of people you want contact with and extend it when you are feeling a little stronger.

If you are in partnership, this is a couples issue and should be approached as such. Sometimes it is an unenviable position for a partner to be in. One minute they are the spouse, the next they are the carer and when things go wrong, even the cleaner. Try and be patient with one another and talk about the difficulties to accommodate each other in the most supportive way.

Useful tips

As a patient, you come under the scrutiny of all systems and soon realise that no facet of your life will remain untouched.

Here is my to-do list:

- » Call for a family meeting and share the findings, interventions and any concerns you have with them
- » Draw up a will or update your existing one
- » Draw up a living will if you deem this necessary
- » Put your house in order
- » Keep ongoing records of your interventions
- » Keep a journal of your experiences
- » Do not bring valuables to the hospital
- » Make sure you bring your identity document, your medical aid details and your procedure codes
- » Bring a list of your medications and their dosages
- » Alert staff to allergies
- » Educate yourself about the procedure
- » Educate yourself about the inherent risks involved in the surgery, both short and long term
- » Alert the anaesthetist to any complications during previous surgery
- » Choose a unit with a multi-disciplinary approach and, if possible, is research-based, to ensure that the team is up-to-date with the latest findings in the field
- » Choose surgeons who are well thought of by their colleagues, and have the experience required in this specific area of surgery
- » Do not undergo surgery at a time when the attending physician is about to go on leave
- » Make sure the staff have familiarised you with the necessary pre-operative preparation
- » Ensure that you understand that you will probably recover in ICU and what this entails

- Decide in advance who will accompany you to hospital and who you would like to visit you while in hospital. Screen your visitors well
- Draw up a list of your requirements for your week-long stay on the ward
- If you have any questions that need answering prior to surgery, write them down and discuss them with your surgeon
- Don't take a long book like *War and Peace* by Dostoyevsky. Your concentration post-surgery will be greatly compromised, so magazines with pictures should do the trick
- Attend to all arrangements related to the running of the home in your absence and delegate, delegate, delegate
- Relinquish the mother role until you have recuperated and then take it up on advisement!
- Remember, you are the patient. The rest of the family need to take care of themselves and you because you have enough on your plate.

Patient screening

Firstly, let it be said that when you need surgery you need surgery. Screening a patient does not mean that you will be turned away from treatment. Screening is done in the interests of the patient and their subsequent recovery.

The medical background report may serve as an indicator of areas that may be problematic, for example the bio-psychosocial and sexual concerns that you (and your partner) may be facing.

Psychological screening should be carried out by someone who is both familiar with the field and has a particular interest in women's health. Psychological screening allows for the correct interventions to be put in place to support you both prior and post-surgery.

Support should also be provided if indicated or requested. If your profile reflects a history of depression, anxiety, a troubled childhood and trauma, you should request additional support. A number of validated depression, anxiety, hostility, and somatisation scales are available to ascertain psychological concerns facing women undergoing this kind of surgery.

Pre-operative support wish-list

» Patients in distress have selective hearing. For this reason, doctors should place special emphasis on clarifying what the nature of the problem is and which surgery is indicated.

» Reading material should be provided for patients to read when they return home, or refer them to an informative website linked to the unit.

» Husbands or partners should be included in a similar orientation to clarify the nature of the problem and the required intervention.

» A seminar for patients about to undergo specific surgery may prove beneficial to clarify concerns, provide support and lessen the patients' feelings of isolation.

» It is important to address concerns related to patient expectations, and goals related to the surgery.

» Support structures need to be put in place to manage the emotional aspects of the procedure from admission to hospitalisation to aftercare and follow-up.

» An opportunity should be made available to couples and patients who express concern regarding the impact the surgery may have on their sexual functioning, intimacy and relationship.

Post-operative support

Indicators for concern post-surgery

» Compaction (severe, immovable constipation)
» Bladder infection (fever and a burning sensation when passing urine)
» Wound infection
» Vaginal or wound bleeding
» Vault haematoma
» Bright red fresh blood following a mesh insertion may be indicative of the mesh perforating the vaginal wall and would indicate removal of the mesh
» Pain and swelling in the legs impacting on weight-bearing may be indicative of a deep vein thrombosis and should be attended to immediately

If there is a hotline for patients this would prove to be most useful. In this instance, the nursing sister attached to the colorectal or pelvic floor unit will decide, in consultation with the surgeon, what the next move should be. Should an admission be indicated, it is advisable that you be admitted to the hospital where the initial surgery was done.

Pain

Some patients suffer moderate pain that decreases over time and doesn't return. Others suffer severe pain that comes and goes. Still others suffer various kinds of pain in various places at different times.

Pain can be acute, in which case it is sharp and urgent, but responds to medication. Or it can be chronic, in which case it is ongoing and often needs adjustments to medication and alternate therapies. In fact, chronic pain needs to be managed rather than treated.

Don't be afraid to tell your surgeon or physician about the pain you're in. To help them help you, it's best to examine and analyse the pain you're in before approaching anyone to help you deal with it. Ask and answer these questions:

» Is the pain a dull ache, a burning sensation, a stabbing pain? Describe exactly what it feels like.
» Is the pain in one place, for instance, your lower abdomen, or does it spread to other areas?
» Is the pain constant? If not, when does it occur? Are there times when you're totally pain-free?

If the pain doesn't subside within a reasonable time, keep a daily pain journal. Describe what you were doing when the pain started or got worse. Describe what you did to reduce the pain. Refer to your journal when telling your doctor that you need help with the pain.

Pain control and side effects

Every effort will be made to ensure that pain control is attended to during your hospital stay. The nature of the pain will be discomfort in the lower abdomen.

In the event of abdominal surgery, there will be added discomfort when moving owing to the extensive nature of the surgery. It is important to alert the nursing staff should your pain levels not be responding to the pain medication you're being given.

On discharge, you are provided with painkillers that may cause drowsiness and/or constipation. Constipation is contra-indicated, so it is advisable to see a dietician prior to discharge, who can advise you on the types of food to eat and foods that should be avoided during the recovery period.

To avoid constipation caused by the ongoing use of pain medication containing codeine or dihydrocodeine, eat as much fruit and fibre as possible. Within reason, being active in small bouts will ensure that your strength returns more quickly, which will prevent the formation of blood clots in your legs or lungs.

Body functioning

How your body responds to surgery depends a great deal on what surgery you undergo and how severe your condition is. If your condition is severe, you can expect some changes in the way your body recovers. You may experience incontinence, both urinary and faecal, for which you'll have to make provision.

Speak to your doctor about the long-term effects of the surgery – is the incontinence temporary or permanent? Are there exercises you can do to prevent the condition worsening? Discuss your concerns openly.

Any surgery represents trauma to the physical body. And a body in trauma needs time to recover. Don't expect to be up and running within days or weeks. Give your body the time it needs to heal the wounds of surgery and rebuild its core strength.

Possible post-operative complications

We've already discussed pain as a complication of surgery in the pelvic area and how to identify and manage it. There can be other complications, which many women may never experience. However, if you do suspect that 'something has gone wrong', you need to alert your surgeon immediately.

Complications immediately after surgery can include bowel obstruction, urine leaking, infection and delayed bleeding, which is rare.

Most of the complications that occur months after the surgery involve the mesh. Symptoms include mesh erosion, hardening of the mesh, recurrence of the type of pain and discomfort you experienced before the surgery, serious infection, vaginal discharge, urinary problems and painful intercourse.

Changes in sexual functioning and intimacy

Initially sexual intercourse may be sensitive; however, this should settle down after three months. Should the vaginal narrowing not allow for penetration post-surgery, consult your surgeon. This may be surgically rectified, although the procedure is complex. Referral to a sex therapist, if indicated, should be arranged to address any sexual related queries and concerns related to this area.

Topics such as sexual contact, non-genital stimulation and different positions for intercourse should be addressed if relevant.

Monthly couples sessions to address couples' concerns post-surgery may prove to be most beneficial. Written material is helpful because it allows patients to review what has been discussed in the comfort of their homes.

Emotional support

Pelvic floor surgery is often major surgery that lasts for hours and leaves you and your body traumatised. This is not the time to surround yourself with cheerleaders who need you to recover quickly or family members who are convinced you did this to yourself and are lapping up the sympathy. This is also not the time to keep everything to yourself because you've had surgery in 'unmentionable places'.

If you aren't surrounded by people who love, care about and respect you, and you feel the need to talk to women who have been through similar experiences, find a support group or go into therapy with a female psychologist who focuses on women's issues. Simply telling your story and having it witnessed by an outsider is remarkably healing.

If you're married or in a partnership, it is a good idea to involve your partner in your recovery. Issues of diminished sexual intimacy, and your diminished capacity to socialise or even help around the house, can become major issues when not addressed.

Make a list of questions and concerns before your sessions so that you don't arrive home realising you forgot to ask about something that troubles you. Your concerns may be purely practical or may be emotional or spiritual. As this book illustrates, pelvic floor prolapse triggers intense emotions at times. Don't ignore these emotions hoping they'll go away on their own. Sustained emotional stress, when not expressed, plays itself out in the body. This prevents whole healing.

Guidelines for healthcare practitioners

Without being presumptuous, certain things do come to mind based on my personal experience and from narratives shared by women in similar situations.

» First and foremost, acknowledge the whole being who seeks your expertise. This is not a health issue, this is a human issue presenting as a health problem.
» Refrain from not listening to and hearing the unique narratives of patients.
» Broaden the lenses through which you view the patient. In addition to asking how often they urinate and defaecate, ask how this impacts on their lives and the lives of their partners.
» Provide referral for appropriate psychological support wherever possible. If patients are unable to afford psychological assistance, refer them to helping professionals who will be willing to negotiate their fees on a sliding scale. Some professionals are willing to dedicate a certain number of hours to pro bono work.
» Always remember that physical and mental health are closely linked and interdependent in the healing process ahead.
» Your time is at a premium, but the importance of keeping up-to-date records and sharing information with the allied professionals you refer patients to remains essential. When

this is compromised, the patient will not receive holistic care. A highly effective multi-disciplinary team where concerns are shared has proved to be the best option for both the patient and the physicians treating them.

» Know that patients are able to form strong bonds with their doctors. To you they may be just another patient, but your significance to them far outweighs this. Honour that through care, concern and compassion.
» Patients should be encouraged to take ownership of their health because if they do not, someone or something else will. Horn (2013:11) emphasises the importance of patients' decisions to take responsibility for their recovery in order to reduce as far as possible the causes of distress that they experience, and where this is not possible, to provide them with the wherewithal to cope as best they can.

CHAPTER TWO

A QUICK WALK THROUGH HOSPITAL AND BACK HOME

Hospital admission

- In most instances, you will be admitted to hospital on the morning of your surgery.
- The surgeon and the anaesthetist will consult with you prior to the surgery to address any concerns you may raise.
- A sedative may be administered to lower your anxiety level.
- The complexity of the surgery will determine the duration of the surgery, the mode (vaginally, abdominally or laparoscopically) and the duration of your hospitalisation.

Admission to the Intensive Care Unit

- Post-surgery, you may be transferred to ICU for 24–48 hours and then returned to the pelvic floor ward.
- While in ICU or High Care you will receive bed baths to ensure that your feel clean and refreshed.

Effects of the anaesthetic

» You may experience drowsiness and possible confusion following surgery, but know that it will be of short duration.
» Once discharged the drowsiness and tiredness may continue for a while, so do regard this as normal.

Post-surgery fluid intake

» Initially a drip inserted into your arm will provide the necessary fluid requirement.
» Additional fluid intake may include sips of water or ice cubes.
» Fluid intake is vital and when appropriate, you will be provided with liquid meals, jelly, custard, tea or a light meal.
» Your drip will be removed when you are able to drink again.

Post-surgery urine drainage and pact removal

» Following surgery, a catheter is often inserted in the bladder to drain the urine for up to 24 hours.
» Should you develop urinary incontinence, know that it can be surgically corrected. Regular fluid intake in the form of water is advisable throughout the day.
» Caffeine drinks are to be avoided, as they tend to cause bladder irritability. Inadequate fluid intake may exacerbate bladder irritability.
» An anterior vaginal repair may change your urine flow so do not be alarmed. You will need to regain full bladder functioning before discharge is considered.
» In the event that a length of gauze, like a large tampon (pact), has been inserted in the vagina to reduce the risk of bleeding, it will be removed once you return to the general ward.

- You can expect to have some vaginal bleeding/discharge for 2 to 3 weeks after surgery, which gradually diminishes over time.
- It is advisable to use sanitary pads and avoid tampons, as this may increase the risk of infection.
- The colour of the discharge is brownish red, but will eventually subside.

Pain control and side effects

- Every effort will be made to ensure that pain control is attended to during your hospital stay.
- The nature of the pain experienced will be discomfort in the lower abdomen.
- In the event of abdominal surgery, there will be added discomfort when moving owing to the extensive nature of the surgery. It is important to alert the nursing staff should your pain levels not be responding to the pain medication.

Post-operative scarring

- Scarring post-surgery is minimal, especially if the surgery is done through the vagina or laparoscopically.
- Dissolvable stitches will not need to be removed.
- Should you require abdominal surgery, the surgical clips used will be removed six weeks' post-surgery by your general practitioner or surgeon.
- Abdominal scarring will be more marked but will fade with time.

Bed baths and showers

You should be able to take a shower two days after surgery, provided you feel strong enough.

Physiotherapy

- Physiotherapy will commence within 24 hours following surgery and will continue during the hospitalisation period.
- Early mobility post-surgery will decrease the incidence of developing deep vein thrombosis.
- To avoid clots reaching the lungs (pulmonary embolism), you will receive daily injections of a blood-thinning agent and will need to wear compression stockings until your mobility has significantly improved.
- Special mechanical boots attached to your lower legs will inflate and deflate at periodic intervals to prevent deep vein thrombosis (DVT) while in hospital.
- Your body has been through major surgery, so consult a physiotherapist who will instruct you on pelvic floor exercises to strengthen the pelvic floor. The sooner the core muscles are strengthened the easier the recovery will be.
- The physiotherapist will advise you on exercises to be done during your stay in hospital as well as when you return home.

Dietetics

- It is important that you see a dietician in hospital to guide you on what you should and should not eat after surgery.
- With regular bowel movements a high priority and constipation contraindicated, high-fibre diets are the most suitable option.

Hospital visitors

- Manage hospital visits by family in accordance with how you are feeling.
- Children are not allowed to visit in the wards after surgery, so inquire what the hospital policy is in this regard.

Factors impacting on recovery

- The complexity of the surgery may require a longer recovery period, as is the case with any abdominal surgery.
- Patients suffering from depression or diabetes may experience a more complicated recovery.
- Diabetes, smoking and being overweight are known causes of slowing down the healing process.

Indicators for concern post-surgery

- Additional concerns may include compaction.
- To avoid constipation caused by the ongoing use of pain medication containing codeine or dihydrocodeine, eat as much fruit and fibre as possible. Within reason, being active in short bouts enables your strength to return more quickly and prevents the formation of blood clots in the legs or lungs.
- Additional concerns include bladder infection, wound infection, vaginal or wound bleeding, vault haematoma[47], bright-red fresh blood following a mesh insertion, and pain and swelling in the legs.

Additional protective measures once discharged

- Make sure that you rest sufficiently.
- Make use of existing supports within the family system. Contact your surgeon should you have cause for concern.
- Diligently attend your post-operative appointments and make a list of all concerns you wish to raise prior to the consultation.
- Continue to reconnect with friends and family as your strength increases in order to avoid becoming isolated.

---

47 A blood clot at the top of the vagina

- Set realistic short-term goals in order to reintegrate back into the life you knew prior to surgery.
- Do not undertake physical exercises or any physical activity that will put undue strain on your pelvis in order to ensure optimal post-surgery recovery.
- The sooner the core muscles are strengthened, the easier the recovery will be. But do not rush the process.
- The best forms of exercise are swimming and walking at least 30 minutes a day.
- Start off slowly initially and build your strength up gradually, as this will assist in the healing process.
- Be alert to any change in pain levels and bodily symptoms that you experience as out of the ordinary and seek immediate help.
- You may experience discomfort or pain when standing or sitting for any length of time, make sure that you do not exert yourself.
- Each patient's resilience and strength is different and you need to honour your body's need to rest.
- As your pain decreases, mobility will increase and your energy levels will return to normal. Afternoon naps usually prove to be most useful.
- You are advised not to drive for the first six weeks.

Telephonic support

- Once you return home, you can contact a designated nursing sister to answer questions and concerns that may arise at this time.
- She will also serve as a go-between between you and the surgeon.
- Should an admission be indicated, it is advisable that you be admitted to the hospital where the initial surgery was done.

Return of a sense of wellbeing

» By the fourth week, you should be experiencing an increasing sense of wellbeing.
» If there have been no complications, you should be able to return to normal activities and to resume work by the eighth week.
» You need to keep your weight down if you wish for a positive outcome post-surgery. Should you experience any discomfort or dryness, use a vaginal lubricant.
» At your six-week post-operative check-up, you will be well on your way to recovery. Make sure you listen to bodily symptoms and allow yourself to rest when needed.

Traveling out of town

» Check with your surgeon that you are well enough to travel.
» Lengthy aeroplane or car journeys are contraindicated because they increase your risk of DVT, especially soon after surgery.
» Make sure that you take out sufficient travel insurance and that medical assistance is available at your destination, if necessary.

Things to remember

» Should you experience a marked decline in mood, alert your specialist so that you can be referred for supportive intervention, if required.
» Make sure that you continue with your physiotherapy. When you do return to work, do so gradually.
» Look after yourself and remember, Rome was not built in a day.
» View the surgery as a temporary interruption as you slowly recuperate and regain your previous quality of life.

Embrace the questions that surface

The vulnerability that surgery leaves you feeling, the revisiting of that childlike dependent state, may serve as the catalyst for the surfacing of other losses. You have little resilience, you have time on your hands while recuperating, and the dark shadows know this. So when the weariness and vulnerability set in and painful memories from the past surface, know that this is appropriate and let them do so. What you resist persists.

Welcome this period and know that the emotional roller coaster that it may bring in its wake is normal. If it feels like the load is too heavy, talk to a close confidant or seek out a good counsellor. The courage to seek help is far braver than leaving yourself in a downward spiral of negative emotions. Take a leaf out of my book.

Even if your body feels like it's failing you, don't let this detract from your sense of self-worth. Don't let the illness leave you flawed; rather view it as an opportunity to look at the flawed aspects of yourself. So use this as a time for self-reflection and a life review. Find a way to make sense of the experience physically, emotionally and transformatively. Grab every moment, savour life, redefine what you want from life going forward, and fight for the dreams you have. And above all, recommit to life.

When the soul is off track in this lifetime, and patterns in one's life repeat over and over, then it is time to do the work of the unconscious with a view to re-evaluating your relationship to yourself and others, and your relationship to the Divine. We know that deep and hidden wounding causes illness, so we need to seek out the wounding and its causes to start healing the body's wounds. So be sensitive to the whispers from the inner landscape of your body if you wish to participate in the dance of healing.

The challenge is to pay specific attention to all forms of dis-ease within the body and, in doing so, benefit emotionally, spiritually and psychologically.

Women need to focus not on the healing of the condition, but more on the reason why the condition surfaced in the first place. What issues in your life need confronting? Why G-d has shifted you out of complacency through illness if not to urge you to search for healing on all levels?

Healing should be a journey, a process of self-discovery, and the new-born, healthy you should encompass deep inner healing of your mind and spirit. If not, the symptoms will keep knocking at your door, until you heed the call. But answering a call in the depth of the night is a choice, and embarking on a healing journey is also a choice. It rests on the concept of free will and the use of your own Geiger counter.

You have to take responsibility for your healing in every sense of the word, no matter how long the journey, no matter how many obstacles along the way. It requires commitment and passion to search for a better life. You have to name the demon confronting you and take on the challenge with all your being, precisely because no other person can take this responsibility on for you.

This is your journey, your own dark night of the soul.

CHAPTER THREE

HOW TO TRULY CARE FOR HER

In the prelude to this book, I wrote of the deep friendship between Lorraine and me.

From the outset, we have celebrated and learned as much from the similarities between us as the differences. She married and had children; I never did. She studied social sciences; I trained as a nurse and later studied languages. She focused on community; I focused on singular experience. She contemplated human dynamics and traditional Judaism; I contemplated consciousness in a world of form.

We approached life and religion from very different angles and brought to one another ideas and knowledge that meshed as we discussed them. Somehow we always met in the middle.

We met in our early 40s and here in our mid-60s, I have seen her life change from a dynamic interconnected buzz of activity to the fragile cave of isolation in which she now lives. I have felt angry at losing a friend to a relentless illness that allows for very little more than managing each day. I have felt powerless to help or change anything. I have wondered often whether I would have had her courage and fortitude if I were in the same circumstances. I have been afraid of losing her, afraid that this will never come right, afraid that this diminished life is all that is left for her.

Then a year ago, she began to change and grow and rise above it all. She came to understand that the illness was a friend asking her to meet it in the middle. She wondered how many women go through similar trials and how they cope. She began to research pelvic floor dysfunction and found huge gaps in knowledge and very few resources for women with her condition. She decided to address that, and I have my friend back.

Here's what I've learned as someone feeling powerless on the side-lines wondering what on earth they could do to make her life a little easier. As someone who has watched how the people close to her have treated her. I have studied those who remained steadfast by her side and those who fled in some way, even if not physically.

Get over yourself: If you really want to help, become the person who can look past all the gore and see the human struggling to survive. Even when all she can talk about is body functions and pain, muscle weakness and loss of balance, see the soul in experience of a frightening reality.

Let her talk about the tough stuff: If she wants to discuss her death, let her. If she's dumping on herself for all the things she didn't do and all the things she'll never do or be again, let her. Be there in the moment even if it brings up feelings of loss and grief. Be there even if you've heard it all before and are very likely to hear it all again.

Don't allow guilt to enter: You feel like the one who got away. You're healthy and she's seriously ill. You didn't do this to her, you simply witnessed it and are still witnessing it. So what if you've never had an operation yourself and she's heading for her seventh? What does that have to do with the connection between you? What does that have to do with what she needs from you in this moment? It is her connections to others that keep her afloat, that stop her from losing all hope. Sustain and maintain that connection, no matter what.

Don't berate yourself for negative feelings: There are times you'll feel frustrated and desperate because nothing seems to get better. Small wins set you up for huge defeats. And you want to blame her for everything. The time and money all this is costing. The limits placed on your life. All the things you can no longer do together or expect of her. Know that these and a range of other feelings and thoughts are nothing but natural. You're healthy, but her ill health is impacting on your life and the lives of everyone in the system. You know she's not to blame, but you've got to blame someone. None of this feels fair. None of this has a reason you can latch onto. Breathe through all the feelings. Acknowledge that you have the right to feel these things. And come through knowing that when all is said and done, you love this person. And that's the most important thing of all.

Do everything you possibly can to protect her dignity: When she's having a good day, go with it. Don't break her down by telling her all the things you think and feel. Don't criticise her to make yourself feel better. If you need help in this time, go into therapy, learn to dance on a shifting carpet.

Help her cope with the losses: Some of the people in her life when she was well are likely to abandon her. They do this out of fear and ignorance. They don't know how to cope with her. They can't look in the mirror and see that this or something like it could happen to them. They can't watch her run out of money and resources. They can't watch her run out of time. All you need to do is simply be there. She doesn't need spectacular gestures and huge donations of time and money. She needs connection and presence.

Find out every last thing you can about her condition: Simply Google 'pelvic floor dysfunction' and you'll discover a world of pain and shame that you could help alleviate in the life of at least one person. Read up on patient care so that you can anticipate her needs. Read Part 1 of this book if you want to know more about what she's going through. But remember that Lorraine's condition is severe and fraught with complications. Your person might never experience the illness to this degree, but knowing the worst will help you appreciate what is happening now.

Help in practical ways: If she's going for surgery, tests, procedures, find out what she needs to do in preparation and help in any way you can. Help fill in the 10-page medical history form. Buy the toiletries she'll need. Help her pack her suitcase. Remember the dates and times of appointments and make sure she has a way to get there. Think ahead. Plan for the worst, hope for the best. Simple, like that.

Practise on your sainthood: Listen. Be present. Remain connected. Care. Keep the wolves away from her door. And please don't be the wolf at her door.

This isn't about you. This is about other. And we are the ones we love.

REFERENCES

Adahan, Miriam. 1992. *It's All a Gift*. Feldheim Pubishers. Jerusalem.

Alappattu, M.J. and Bishop, M.D. 2011. Psychological Factors in Chronic Pain in Women: Relevance and Application of the Fear-Avoidance Model of Pain. Journal of American Physical Therapy Association. *Physical Therapy*. October: 91(10):1542–1550.

Alperin, M., Ellison, R., Meyn, L. Franlman, E. and Zyczynski, H.M. 2013. Two-year Outcomes after Vaginal Prolapse Reconstruction with Mesh Pelvic Floor Repair. *Female Pelvic Medical Reconstruction Surgery*. March–April: 19(2):72–78.

Alvarez, J., Cvach, K. and Dwyer, P. 2013. Complications in Pelvic Floor Surgery. *Minerva Medica*. February: 65 9(1):53–67.

Arnando, Elisa. 2013. Persistent Pain as a Pathological Entity. 200–208 in *Chronicity, Care and Complexity*. 25–40. Inter-disciplinary Press, United Kingdom.

Barber, D. 2005. Pelvic Floor Distress Inventory – 20 and Pelvic Floor Impact Questionnaire 7. *American Journal of Obstetrics and Gynaecology*. Vol. 193, Issue 1, July: 103–113.

Borysenko, J. 1997. *A Woman's Book of Life: The Biology, Psychology and Spirituality of the Feminine Life Cycle*. Riverhead Books. New York.

Brown, Brene. 2015. *Rising Strong*. Vermillion. London.

Chauvin, C., Chereau, E. Ballester, M. and Darai, E. 2012. Potential Relevance of Pre-operative Quality of Life Questionnaires to Identify Candidates for Surgical Treatment of Genital Prolapse: A Pilot Study. *BMC Urology*.12:9

Davilla, W., Ghoneim, M. and Wexter, S.D. 2006. *Pelvic Floor Dysfunction: A Multi-disciplinary Approach*. Springer – Verlag London Limited.

Ellefsen, Edith. 2013. The Health Within Illness Model to Reconcile Borderlands Between Health and Illness for People Living with Chronic Disease. 41–52 in *Chronicity, Care and Complexity*. 25–40. Inter-disciplinary Press, United Kingdom.

Engler, D., Baranowski, J., Cottrell, A., Elneil, S., Highes, J., Messelink, E.J., Van Ophoven, A., Reisman, Y. and Williams, A.C. de C. 2014. *Guidelines on Chronic Pelvic Pain*. European Association of Urology. April: Chapters 3–11.

Esu, Aide. 2013. Have You Remembered to Take the Coumadin? Life Trajectories and Invisible Work in the Narratives of Coronary Heart Disease Patients in *Chronicity, Care and Complexity*. 147–158. Inter-disciplinary Press, United Kingdom.

Feldner, P.C., Delrop, C.A., Martins, B.S., Castro, R.A., Sartori, M.G., Girao, M.J.B. 2013. Sexual Function after Anterior Vaginal Wall Prolapse Surgery. *Clinics*. Vol.67, 8:1–7

Ford, Debbie. 2003. *The Secret of the Shadow: The Power of Owning Your Own Story*. Harper. San Fransisco.

Frank, Arthur. 1995. *The Wounded Storyteller*. London. University of Chicago Press Ltd.

Frankl, Victor, E. 2004. *Man's Search for Meaning*. Rider. London.

Goffman, Erving. 1986. *STIGMA: Notes on the Management of Spoiled Identity*. Penguin Books Ltd, Harmondsworth, Middlesex, England.

Goldberg, R., Kesmodel, U.S., Gradel, K.O., Kaerlev, L., Norgard, B.M. 2013. Patient Reported Outcome Measure in Women Undergoing Surgery for Urinary Incontinence and Pelvic Floor Prolapse. *International Urogynecological Journal*. July: 24(7):1127–1134.

Government of Nepal Ministry of Health and Population: Department of Health Services. 2013. *Health Related Quality of Life of Women Suffering from Pelvic Floor Prolapse before and 9 to 11 Months after Surgery*.

Greenbaum, Avraham. 1990. *Rebbe Nachman on Suffering*. The Breslov Research Centre. Jerusalem.

Greenwood, M. and Nunn, Peter. 1996. *The Paradox of Healing: Transforming Your Relationship with Illness*. PRION. Great Britain.

Holfish, K.L., Bobvjerg, V.E., Gibson, J. and Steers, W.D. 2002. Patient-centred Goals for Pelvic Floor Dysfunction Surgery. *American Journal of Obstetrics and Gynaecology*. Vol. 187, Issue 1, July: 88–92.

Hollis, James. 1993. *The Middle Passage: From Misery to Meaning in Midlife*. Inner City Books. Canada.

Hollis, James. 1996. *Swamplands of the Soul: New Life in Dismal Places*. Inner City Books, Canada.

Hollis, James. 2005. *Finding Meaning in the Second Half of Life*. Penguin Group. U.S.A.

Hollis, James. 2010. *What Matters Most: Living a More Considered Life*. Gotham Books. U.S.A.

Horn, Danea. 2013. *Chronic Resilience: 10 Sanity Saving Strategies for Women Coping with the Stress of Illness*. Conari Press. Canada.

Judith, Anodea. 1999. *Wheels of Life: A User's Guide to the Chakra System*. Llewellyn Publications, Minnesota, U.S.A.

Kabat-Zinn, Jon. 2005. *Coming to Our Senses: Healing Ourselves and the World Through Mindfulness*. Hyperion. U.S.A.

Kaplan, Gary and Donna Beach. 2014. *Total Recovery: Solving the Mystery of Chronic Pain and Depression*. Penguin Books. United States of America.

Levy, Naomi. 1998. *To Begin Again: Rebuilding Your Life After Bad Things Have Happened*. Harper Collins Publishing. Great Britain.

Mandell, Judy. 1998. *What to Expect in Your Fifties.: A Woman's Guide to Health and Longevity*. A Dell Trade Paperback. Bantam Doubleday Publishing Group, Inc. New York.

Maolli, P.A., Jones, S.J., Meyn, L.A. Zyczynski, H.M. 2003. Risk Factors Associated with Pelvic Floor Disorders in Women Undergoing Surgical Repair. *Journal of Obstetrics and Gynaecology*. May: Vol. 101. Issue 5 5, Part 1:869–874.

Moore, Thomas. 1992. *Care of the Soul*. Piatkus Books. Great Britain.

Martinez, Mario. 2014. *The MindBody Code: How to Change the Beliefs that Limit Your Health, Longevity, and Success*. Sounds True. Boulder, Colorado.

Myss, C. 2009. *Defy Gravity: Healing Beyond the Bounds of Reason*. Hay House Incorporated, New York.

Myss, C. 2013. *Invisible Acts of Power: Personal Choices that Create Miracles*. Simon and Schuster. New York.

Nicholas, M., Malloy, A., Tonkin, L. and Beeston, L. 2011. *Manage Your Pain: Practical and Positive Ways of Adapting to Chronic Pain.* ABC Books. Australia.

Northrupp, Christiane. 1995. *Women's Bodies, Women's Wisdom: The Complete Guide To Women's Health and Wellbeing.* Piaticus. Great Britian.

Novara, G., Galfano, A., Mancini, M., Ficarra, V. and Artibani, W. 2006. Critical Assessment of Pelvic Floor Surgical Reconstruction Outcome. *EAU-EBU update series.* Vol. 4. 202–213.

Nygard, I., Barber, M.D., Burgio, K.L., Kenton, K., Meikle, S., Schaffer, J., S., Pino, C., Whitehead, W.E, Wu, J., Brody, D. 2008. Prevalence of Pelvic Floor Dysfunction in US Women. *JAMA.* September: 300 (11): 1311–1316.

Pereira, M., Figueirdo and Finchman, F.D. 2011. Anxiety, Depression, Traumatic Stress and Quality of Life in Colorectal Cancer and their Partners after Different Treatments: A study with Portuguese Patients and their Partners. *European Journal of Oncology Nursing.* 1–6.

Rabbi Rabinowitz, Chaim Dov. 2001. *Da'ath Sofrim: Torah, Prophets, Sacred Writings: Commentary on the Book of IYOV (Job).* H. Vagshal Publishing Ltd. New York/Jerusalem.

Riss, P.A. 2003. Review article: Problems and Pitfalls in Pelvic Reconstructive Surgery. *RAVVESTN* 72: II-153–156.

Rosenbaum, Elana. 2012. *Being Well Even When You Are Sick.* Shambhala. Boston.

Rothchild, Babette. 2000. *The Body Remembers. The Psychophysiology of Trauma and Trauma Treatment.* W.W. Norton and Company. New York. London

Shapiro, D. 2006. *Your Body Speaks Your Mind.* Sounds True Inc., Canada.

Shealy, N. and Myss, C.M. 1988. *The Creation of Health: The Emotional, Psychological, and Spiritual Responses that Promote Health and Healing.* Stillpoint Publishing. U.S.A.

Shealy, N. and Myss, C.M. 1993. *The Creation of Health: The Emotional, Psychological and Spiritual Responses that Promote Heath and Healing.* Stillpoint Publishing. U.S.A.

Traal, M.J., De Vries, J., Roukema, J.A. and Oudstein, B.L. 2011. Sexual Dysfunction and the Quality of Sexual Life in Patients with Colorectal Cancer: A Systemic Review. *Annals of Oncology.*

Trowbridge, Bob. 1997. *The Hidden Meaning of Illness: Disease as Symbol and Metaphor.* A.R.E. Press. Virginia.

Walsch, Neale Donald. 2009. *When Everything Changes, Change Everything.* Hodder and Stoughton. London.

Wise, David and Anderson, M.D. 2010. *A Headache in the Pelvis: A New Understanding and Treatment for Chronic Pelvic Pain Syndromes.* 6th Edition. National Centre for Pelvic Pain.

Zerman, Dirk-Hendrik, Ishigooka, M., Doggweiker, R. and Schmidt, R.A. 1998. Postoperative Chronic Pain and Bladder Dysfunction: Windup and Neural Plasticity: Do We Need More Neurological Approaches in Pelvic Floor Surgery? *Official Journal of American Urological Association.* Vol. 160, Issue 1:102–105, July.

Made in United States
Troutdale, OR
11/03/2026

56845374R00113